THE FASTED LIFESTYLE

The Complete Guide to Intermittent Fasting

GW00471170

Ben Smith

FOREWORD

Intermittent fasting can be used as a tool to aid your lifestyle, used differently depending on your goals. Like all lifestyle choices, it will not react the same for everyone. For this reason, my exact blueprint is not provided within this book, although mine is woven in-between the lines. It's up to you to find yours with the information provided, should you wish to try it.

The fasted lifestyle is a product of nearly four years of personal experience with Intermittent Fasting. Not only have I buried myself into the research, but I've also learnt first-hand, making countless mistakes along the way, so you don't have to. This book stems from a place of passion and complete trust and belief in the process. To me, intermittent fasting isn't a quick fix or fad, nor is the sole outcome focused on body composition. It's a tool that can improve the overall quality of one's life.

So, what will you find in the following pages? Like many areas of health and fitness, intermittent fasting is often either over-simplified or over-complicated – it seems to be human nature for us to overshoot one way or the other! My aim with this book is to provide the necessary depth to fully understand the process of fasting and the inter-workings

ABOUT THE AUTHOR

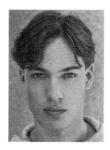

Ben Smith has an Internationally Accredited Diploma in Nutrition and studies Mechanical Engineering at the University of Manchester. In 2016 he rowed at an International level for England, having won numerous national medals prior, before leaving rowing behind due to a string of bad health. His focus turned from fitness to nutrition as a means of finding good health, and a passion for cooking quickly developed - at which point he set up bensmithlive.com. Ben later suffered from IBS as a result of mis-prescribed antibiotics and dedicated his full energy to untangling the field of gut health, as doctors stated there was nothing that could be done. Through nutrition and lifestyle changes alone, Ben is now IBS and health issues free and aims to spread the knowledge gained through his adversity in the hope that it reaches those that might need it.

behind it, such that you can practice it effectively, without needless complication. Should you wish to find out more, then this book can act as a gateway, covering the core understanding so that further research and experimentation can be done.

At times, this book may seem to dive a little deep into the science of how and why fasting works in the way it does. The reason for this is because, in my opinion, the process is best practiced with a complete understanding of what is actually going on below the surface. The current knowledge and research of fasting is also ever-growing; as such, I have based this book on the current research that is present, which is likely to expand in the future.

You and everyone else fasts every night, many break this fast with "break-fast"

CONTENTS

ONE

INTRODUCTION TO INTERMITTENT FASTING

TWO

HOW FASTING WORKS

THREE

HOW TO FAST

FOUR

FASTING CONSIDERATIONS

ONE

INTRODUCTION TO INTERMITTENT FASTING

WHAT IS INTERMITTENT FASTING?

THE HISTORY OF FASTING

THE BENEFITS OF FASTING

WHAT IS INTERMITTENT FASTING?

The type of fasting described in this book is known as time-restricted feeding. Put simply, consuming all of your calories in a given window of the day, usually 8 hours or less, and abstaining from calories in the remaining hours. When you start consuming calories, you push the first domino in a series of responses that allow your body to process what you're consuming, including rising levels of insulin, which converts the food you're consuming into energy, ready to be used or stored for later. The idea of fasting is to restrict this response to a small window of the day, and in doing so, your body will simply use what it already has at its disposal in the remaining hours. What comes with this is a host of physiological, psychological and lifestyle benefits, all of which we'll get to shortly. In the absence of incoming calories, your body also has the opportunity to look internally, processing, prioritising, and removing what is weaker or least vital to it, hence its use for natural healing.

> *"Our food should be our medicine. Our medicine should be our food. But to eat when you are sick is to feed your sickness."*
> *– Hippocrates, widely considered the father of medicine.*

THE FASTED LIFESTYLE

Consuming Nothing vs. Consuming a Small Amount

There is a very big difference between consuming nothing, fasting, and eating a small amount. This idea first became apparent in the mid-1900s, when these two cases were put to the test, albeit at the extreme. The first is the Minnesota Starvation Experiment, where researchers aimed to better understand the effects of hunger and starvation to help people rehabilitate and recover from starvation that resulted from World War II. 36 men consumed 3,200 calories for 3 months, followed by 1,570 calories for 6 months, these figures adjusted to their weight with the aim of losing 1.1kg per week. Participants saw a significant reduction in strength and endurance, body temperature, heart rate and sex drive. Reports claimed that the men would dream, read and talk about food, also displaying fatigue, irritability, and symptoms of depression.[1]

By contrast is the story of Angus Barbieri, who carried out the longest fast recorded to date in 1965, lasting 380 days. Angus started this fast over 200kg in weight, losing a staggering 125kg in the year-long period, consuming no calories whatsoever. This process was carefully monitored with frequent hospital visits and regular blood tests. The report states, "The patient remained symptom-free, felt well and walked about normally," and "prolonged fasting had no ill effects.". Angus' weight also remained stable for years following the fast.[2] The procedural measures of these two studies were far from similar, with Angus being a single individual who initially weighed over 200kg; however, these cases sparked a great debate on the difference between eating nothing and eating not quite enough. So, what causes this contrast?

Making the Metabolic Switch

As I'll explain at length in the upcoming chapters, when you consume regular meals, you keep insulin steadily high, and in doing so, you are unable to access stored fat for energy. You give yourself 'just enough' to keep your metabolism primed for burning glucose as a source of fuel, this glucose being in limited supply - in the case of the study, just a portion of the 1,570 calories consumed. In contrast, by eating nothing, you make the switch from using glucose as a source of fuel to ketones from fat stores, with fat stores being in much greater supply - the average human carrying over 70,000 calories worth of fat on their body.

A finding that may surprise you from Angus' 380-day fast was that blood glucose levels remained consistent at around 30 mg/100 ml for the duration[2], despite no consumption of carbohydrates… How could this be possible? In the absence of incoming carbohydrates, your liver is actually capable of producing glucose from glycerol, which is produced from the breakdown of stored fat. This process is called gluconeogenesis, translating to "making new glucose".

Making the metabolic switch from using glucose as a source of fuel to fatty acids and ketone bodies takes around 8-12 hours after consuming calories, this is the 'post-absorptive range'. Entering what is deemed a 'true fasted state' requires abstaining from incoming calories for some time beyond this range, hence why fasting protocols usually start at 16 hours of fasting, as this is where the beneficial factors really kick in. This metabolic switch has the potential to not just improve body composition but also slow the process of aging and disease development.[3]

Having what is called 'metabolic flexibility' means that our body is able to use glucose and fat at the appropriate times. This is to ensure we enter the most efficient metabolic state based on food availability, so, during the day, we are primed to use glucose as we consume food, and then in the evening, we steer towards using fat. As you'll discover later in 'Gut Health', our gut microbiome ramps up during the day to support the consumption of food and winds down at night. Intermittent fasting also allows you to, almost, 'practice' tapping in and out of the different energy stores, making you much more metabolically flexible. This has been a practiced method for endurance athletes for some time, using fasting or fasted training to practice using both energy sources so that when the lengthy training session or race arrives, they have the greatest access to both energy sources!

> *"Fasting is the greatest remedy – the physician within."*
> *– Benjamin Franklin*

Food for Thought

Your whole life, you've been told that "Breakfast is the most important meal of the day!" But what if it's not? Did you know this phrase was first used by Kellogg's? One of the largest breakfast companies in the world. Just food for thought…

Extended Fasting

I think it's vitally important to understand what happens on a larger scale, so you can better understand what happens in a period of fasting. Take someone who fasts for 5, 10, 15, 30 days perhaps; what happens?

First of all, you can certainly survive. In the absence of incoming food, your body looks internally, metabolising for energy. Starting with glucose as the primary fuel source, moving to fat once the finite stored glycogen has been used. You may wonder where muscle comes into the picture? Or leaves the picture... In short, it doesn't. Muscle tissue has been shown to stick around over extended periods of fasting. I've covered this point comprehensively in the 'Muscle' section.

Over the course of an extended fast, your body initiates a process called cellular autophagy, the death and recycling of the weaker cells in your body. Autophagy is the Greek word for 'self-eating'. Sounds a bit gruesome, I know; just picture it like a self-clean out of all the unnecessary or damaged cells and proteins. This is coupled with a host of other physiological responses, which we will discuss at length in the following chapters.

It may surprise you what happens to hunger levels over the course of an extended fast. Hunger is not as simple as many boil it down to be; it's not a case of the less you eat, the hungrier you get. In fact, extended periods of fasting decrease your overall levels of ghrelin, which controls your hunger signals. So, over time, you actually get less and less hungry, providing you don't eat.[4] What's more, in the initial stages of a fast, you only get hungry at your expected mealtimes, after which the feeling subsides altogether.

Many have turned to extended fasting as a cure for a range of chronic illnesses and pains, finding that when put in a fasted state, the body has the ability to eradicate what threatens it. In fact, there's a very long history of fasting for healing. Do note, extended fasting is a different ball game to what I'm discussing and requires a very different approach, producing different effects. I'm not advising fasting to such lengths here, merely using it as an example.

"In a fast, the body tears down its defective parts and then builds anew when eating is resumed."
– Herbert M. Shelton

THE HISTORY OF FASTING

The Evolutionary Standpoint – When Fasting Was Involuntary

Prior to the time when food was readily available, humans had no choice but to go extended periods of time without food. If they weren't able to function in these times, they simply wouldn't have survived. Do bear in mind this isn't a distant memory in the grand scheme of human history. The hunter-gatherer culture can be dated back as far as 2 million years ago, and until roughly 12,000 years ago, all humans still practiced hunter-gathering. One could argue that having required far less frequent food for such a long period of time, that our bodies are not adapted to such a high meal frequency, all with snacks in between. It also stands to reason that having required the ability to hunt for extended periods of time, without continuous food, that we as humans are evolutionarily designed to function at a high level in the absence of incoming food.

I know what you're thinking, and yes, food is readily available, and the challenges of the modern world are not the same as for hunter-gatherers. There is a huge difference between involuntary and voluntary fasting, especially psychologically. Abstaining from food when you have no choice is very different to resisting the overwhelming temptations of modern food culture, a culture that I myself unapologetically love. The good news is, you don't have to choose! The idea of intermittent fasting is that you can enjoy the benefits of both. In an upcoming chapter, 'Modern Day Fasting', I address this disparity and discuss how you can stack the odds in your favour to make involuntary fasting natural in what has become an unnatural environment for it!

> *"The ability to function at a high level, both physically and mentally, during extended periods without food may have been of fundamental importance in our evolutionary history."*
> *– Mattson et al., 2014*

Replacing the Involuntary with Voluntary

Fasting is the most deeply rooted medical practice in history. As food became more abundant, many ancient cultures replaced the involuntary fasted periods with voluntary periods of fasting. One example is the Ancient Greeks, who referred to fasting as times of cleansing, detoxification or purification. In the words of Plutarch, Greek writer and philosopher, "Instead of using medicine, rather, fast for a day.".

Fasting continues to be a deeply rooted part of nearly all religions; in fact, the healing power of fasting was a shared idealism of Jesus Christ, the Prophet Muhammad and Buddha. Judaism has several annual fasts, Muslims fast during the month of Ramadan, Christians fast during Lent, the list really does go on... Many of these practices also emphasise self-discipline, sacrifice, empathy and wisdom.

More recently, through the late 20th century, the idea of eating outside of your mealtimes was a foreign concept. Do your grandparents eat a meal outside of breakfast, lunch or dinner? Maybe here and there but likely not 5 meals a day, all with snacks in-between! The choice of coming home from school and sticking a meal in the microwave certainly wasn't an option when they were young. Although not fasting per se, this speaks volumes of the recent rise in meal frequency.

So, what happened? In short, the practice of fasting has become extinct with rising food availability and consumerism. Food companies now aim to heighten your senses, tempting with mouth-watering advertisements, marketing techniques and highly palatable foods. If abstaining from food, the odds certainly aren't in your favour. How to unstack these odds? We'll get to that shortly.

> *"The principle of fasting is taught in almost all major world religions as a means of developing a higher level of self-mastery and self-control, and also a deeper awareness of how really dependent we are."*
> *– Stephen Covey*

THE BENEFITS OF FASTING

Which of these benefits attract your eye will be personal. Some will apply to you, some might not, others I may have left off that you discover for yourself! The common theme, however, is that they can all improve one's quality of life. A point to note, the way that you fast may impact which of these benefits you experience and also to what extent. All may occur.

Biological

Can facilitate fat loss and muscle gain - Not a given, of course; however, these are facilitated by many of the benefits of fasting listed below and points that will be discussed at great depth in the coming chapters.

Lower overall insulin levels[5] - Having too much insulin can lead to a whole host of health problems. Low levels also increase leptin and hormone-sensitive lipase.

Increases insulin sensitivity[6] - This means your body uses glucose more effectively; this stabilises blood sugar levels.

Reduces oxidative stress[6] - Oxidative stress is an imbalance between the free radicals and antioxidants in the body, both produced naturally by cells. Free radicals can arise from lots of things, spanning from psychological stress to industrial vegetable oils (especially when heated).

Increases human growth hormone[7] - Human growth hormone aids in maintaining lean mass and also healthy tissue in the brain. It's also clinically associated with having a greater lean body mass and a lower body fat percentage.

Reduces inflammation[8] - Decreasing inflammation in your body has great long-term health benefits, also combating joint pain and soreness! For me, a lack of soreness resulting from training has been a hugely noticeable benefit.

Promotes cellular autophagy[9] - Cellular autophagy is the death, recycling and excretion of weaker cells in your body. Your body looks internally, processing and prioritising, discarding weaker cells in the body.

Improves cognition and brain function[3] - Cognition is your ability to think, understand, learn and perceive. Intermittent fasting stimulates BDNF, which plays a major role in both memory and learning.

Improves blood cholesterol profile[10] - High blood cholesterol is associated with health issues including cardiovascular disease, high blood pressure and diabetes.

Greater fat mobilisation and fatty acid oxidation[11] - This means that your body is more effective at breaking down fat and using it for energy whilst fasting.

Increases metabolism or mitigates the fall resulting from weight loss[12] - Fasting has been shown to maintain or even increase resting energy expenditure and can also mitigate the fall in metabolism that results from weight loss, ensuring you stay sharp, even if you're losing weight.

Improves digestion - Intermittent fasting gives your digestive system the time it needs to rest, digest and heal if necessary – this is the case for digestive issues such as leaky gut.

Strong ties to increased longevity[13] - Longevity literally means how long you live - this research is still early in development.

Allows your gut flora to thrive[14] - Intermittent fasting can improve the diversity of the microbes in the gut, also helping to fend off those that are less wanted.

Clearer skin - A product of reduced inflammation, improved gut flora and more, conditions such as acne and eczema may improve.

Re-associate yourself with hunger and learning to control it - Hunger is a natural and necessary process, but at times, it can be difficult to manage. Getting a handle on hunger can hugely impact one's day-to-day life.

Protection against neurodegenerative diseases such as Alzheimer's and Parkinson's[3] - A multitude of studies dating back over a century suggest that fasting can have preventative effects against a number of diseases.

Lifestyle

Increases productivity - When food isn't a choice until later in the day, your mind is free to focus on the task at hand. This is especially the case when coupled with stable energy levels and improved cognition.

Easier to find a calorie deficit - For those seeking specific goals that require a calorie deficit, decreasing the time window in which you eat makes this much easier to achieve.

Reduces decision fatigue - Willpower is like a muscle; it can only be worked so hard. Reducing decisions that you make on what you consume means your mental energy can be spared for other areas of life.

Lack of bloating - With optimal digestion, you can keep bloating at bay. With reduced meal frequency, you may also reduce the need to rush eating, especially in the morning hurry out the door.

Saves money - Naturally, less money may be spent on food, especially when away from home.

Less time preparing food and everything that comes with it - Choosing what to eat, cooking, eating, cleaning, waiting for the food to go down...

Adds structure to your day - This is especially the case should you choose to fast until the same time every day or on the same days every week. Structure plays a key role in productivity.

Builds a better understanding of the psychology of eating - Once you understand how the body reacts without food, it puts into perspective the psychological influence of eating.

Helps with jetlag - Meal timing is an important signal in regulating our circadian rhythm. Having a regular marker for when you eat can ease the transition into a new time zone.

Say goodbye to tracking! For some... - If you do not have strict goals, your tracking days may be over. And even if you are still tracking, you'll have far less frequent meals to track!

Improves sleep quality - This is personal and depends on how you fast, especially the duration. Many, like myself, see a vast improvement in sleep quality. You may also find you start to dream more!

TWO

HOW FASTING WORKS

MUSCLE – WHY FASTING DOESN'T BURN IT

HOW WE MAINTAIN ENERGY IN THE ABSENSE OF FOOD

COGNITION – WHAT IS IT? HOW AND WHY DOES FASTING IMPROVE IT?

HUNGER AND HOW TO KEEP A LID ON IT

AN EFFECTIVE WEIGHT LOSS STRATEGY THAT PROTECTS YOUR METABOLISM

FASTING FOR GUT HEALTH

STRESS – THE GOOD AND THE BAD

THE FASTED LIFESTYLE

MUSCLE – WHY FASTING DOESN'T BURN IT

A common myth is that fasting causes you to burn muscle, and this point may take some convincing, but I will address that here... The human body has evolved to store energy as glycogen and body fat and to use it when required. So, when you require energy in the absence of incoming food, your body will naturally use these two pathways that are designed to supply you with just that. Muscle tissue, on the other hand, is not designed to supply you with energy; it's vital functional tissue that the body acts to preserve.

Still not quite convinced? A real-world study showed that alternate day fasting, only eating every other day, for 70 days caused an 11.4% decrease in fat mass, whilst lean mass (muscle and bone) didn't change at all. Like I've said previously, in the absence of food, your body processes and prioritises, discarding what is least vital. Your lean muscle is vital, hence why your body has systems in place primed to protect it.

How does this happen? There are a number of physiological responses that seem to make this possible, including a rise in counter-regulatory hormones, such as human growth hormone (HGH).[7] Again, not terms to shy away from, a completely natural response. Nørrelund and colleagues put this idea to the test in a 2001 study, where fasted subjects took an HGH suppressant to see the subsequent outcome on muscle breakdown. Suppressing HGH led to a staggering 50% increase in muscle breakdown, highly suggesting that human growth hormone plays a critical role in the preservation of muscle during fasting.[16]

So, where is muscle lost? By not providing your body with a reason to keep it, through the correct stimulus, or training, chronically cutting your calories aside. By sending the right signals to your body, through exercise and training stimulus, it's almost like saying, "I need those, better keep them around". Now, of course, it's much more complex than this; just remember that the human body is highly adaptive and will adapt to the workload that you give it over time. A very simple, and some might say, "Bro-science" way to visualise this is that your body is a reflection of the inputs that you feed into it. If a muscle is being worked with continued or increasing weight and volume, you supply it with the stimulus, or reason, to respond accordingly by sticking around or growing. Likewise, if you stop training, you're no longer providing the muscle a reason to stick around, so it will adjust accordingly to this new workload.

The key takeaway here is that during the fasted period, due to responses including rising human growth hormone, your body will preserve lean muscle tissue. Do note that optimising muscle growth is an entirely different discussion. Yes, the food you consume and the quantity of it will directly affect your ability to perform and recover, and subsequently gain muscle, no doubt about it. The point of focus here is that your hard-earned muscle isn't going to drip away during those intermittent periods of fasting. In fact! That human growth hormone response will only cater to muscular development should you feed yourself sufficiently between the fasted periods.

A final note: This has its limitations; extended periods of fasting, very low body weight or body fat and chronically cutting your calories in the periods where you are eating may start to burn muscle tissue.

Hugh Jackman uses intermittent fasting to pack on lean muscle for movies, starting with 'Wolverine' in 2013.

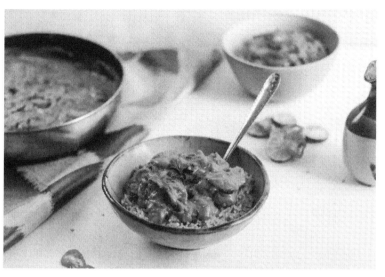

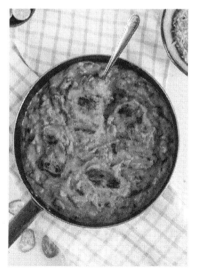

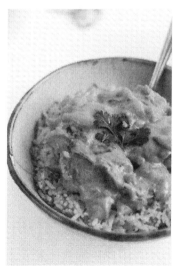

SATAY CHICKEN THIGHS WITH PILAU RICE – SERVES 4

Ingredients:

1 butternut squash (or sweet potato)
2 tbsps nut butter of choice (peanut, almond, etc.)
125ml water
1 tbsp coconut oil
3 white onions
3 cloves of garlic
1 thumb of ginger
1 red chilli or a tsp flakes
½ tbsp red curry paste and additional to taste
8 chicken thighs (alternative: cooked lentils)
2 courgettes
2 red peppers
1 aubergine
250g rice
750ml water
1 tsp turmeric
1 tsp cumin seeds
1 tsp cardamom pods
3-4 bay leaves
Crack of salt
½ lemon juice
1 tsp ground coriander
Crack of salt and pepper

Method:

1. Precook butternut squash (or sweet potato) by peeling, seeding and chopping before roasting in the oven for 25 minutes, or microwaving in a contained dish with a splash of water to steam for 7 minutes.

2. Blend butternut squash, nut butter of choice (almond) and water to create a thick liquid base for later use.

3. In a large frying pan or pot, on a medium-high heat, fry onions, garlic, ginger, chilli and red curry paste with coconut oil until onions start to brown.

4. Add the chicken thighs to the pan and cook until the outsides are seared – this will take 5-10 minutes.

5. Add courgette, red peppers and aubergines with a 1/4 of the blended squash mixture. Cover and continue cooking for 10-15 mins or until the vegetables are almost cooked.

6. Add rice, water, turmeric, cumin seeds, cardamom pods and bay leaves to a saucepan with a crack of salt and bring to the boil before reducing to a gentle simmer for 10 minutes – keep an eye on the rice and add a splash of water if it should need it throughout the cooking.

7. Add the remaining blended mixture to the pan, along with lemon juice and ground coriander, cover and continue cooking for 10 minutes whilst the rice cooks.

8. Season with salt and pepper to taste.

9. OPTIONAL: Stir through coconut milk (milder) or additional red Thai paste (hotter) to your preferred taste and consistency.

10. Turn off the heat and leave for a few minutes to thicken.

11. Serve with your simple pilau rice and enjoy!

HOW WE MAINTAIN ENERGY IN THE ABSENCE OF FOOD

The first question to many people's mind: "How do I have energy without consuming food?". The first thing to recognise is that feeling hungry doesn't always mean you need food energy. The best way I can describe this is through an example. If one night you let the rope go a little, let's say it's the Christmas period, and you feast until your heart's content. The next day, regardless of how much you ate, you will still get hungry. Did all of that food energy disappear? No. It's still there waiting to be used… Hunger arises in a cyclical nature at your expected mealtimes.

Now, it doesn't take feasting for you to wake up with energy to spare. On average, glycogen stores take roughly 24 hours to run out.[17] So, once you lose this mental association and adapt to no longer 'expecting' food in a certain period of the day, say the morning, you simply allow your body to use its stored energy. So, should you provide your body with the nutrients it needs while you are eating, the day prior, it's going to be bottled up, ready to be used when you need it.

Secondly, glucose isn't the body's sole source of energy! Fat stores, the body's secondary source of energy, are also waiting in the back. Using a great analogy by Dr Jason Fung & Jimmy Moore, glycogen stores are like the fridge, always accessible and easy to dive into. Fat stores are like the freezer, except the freezer has a padlock on it, which can't be opened unless insulin is suitably low. The more you pry open and use the freezer, the better at it you become. You don't even have to empty the fridge first! Now, what does this mean? To keep it short and sweet, fat stores can't be accessed if insulin is high, fasting reduces insulin, so while you fast, you can access stored fat. Over time, you become better at using this stored fat, even when glycogen stores aren't necessarily low!

And it still doesn't stop there; the sheer process of abstaining from food sets off a series of hormonal responses, including the activation of the sympathetic nervous system, adrenalin and noradrenalin, cortisol and human growth hormone. With increased levels of these counter-regulatory hormones, energy expenditure rises.[8] These words might seem scary, but they're simply the body's natural response to ensure you continue functioning at your best.

To summarise, stable blood sugar is one of the most sought-after benefits of fasting. Gone are the days of the spikes and crashes in energy throughout your day. The more you allow your body to tap into stored energy, the better you become at doing it. With open access to the fridge and freezer, you never have to look for a quick sugar fix because it's all there, waiting to be used...

A Word on Digestion

Digestion of food requires a lot of blood flow and energy, invested energy, which isn't returned until the digestion process is over. We all know a good carb crash or food coma; this is a perfect example of energy used towards digestion, overwhelming your energy supply. When fasting, in the absence of incoming calories, your body's attention is fully focussed on functioning. Not only this but once you do start to eat, you're far more sensitive to what you're consuming as a product of improved insulin sensitivity!

> *"Fasting is the first principle of medicine; fast and see the strength of the spirit reveal itself."*
> - *Rumi*

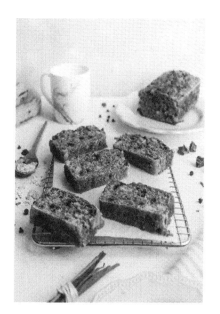

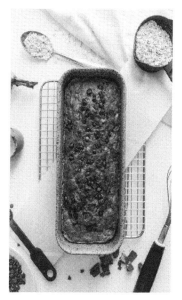

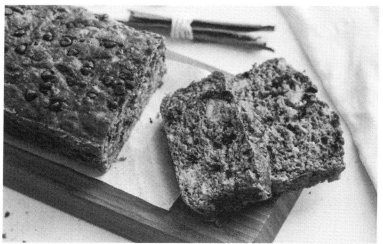

CHOCOLATE CHIP OAT BANANA BREAD

Ingredients:

2 eggs

115g 0% fat Greek yogurt (firm as opposed to runny ie., FAGE)

2 ripe bananas, mashed (250g)

3 tsps maple syrup (grade A)

1tsp vanilla extract

60g rolled oats

1tsp baking soda (bicarbonate of soda)

1 tbsp cinnamon

130g plain white flour

12g cacao nibs or chocolate chips (alternative: broken chocolate pieces)

OPTIONAL: Broken nuts, such as walnuts – fold in with the chocolate

Method:

1. Preheat oven to 180°C and grease your baking tin of choice - I used an 8x4 loaf tin. Alternatively, you can use baking/greaseproof paper.
2. In a mixing bowl, lightly beat the eggs until the yolks are broken.
3. Whisk in the yogurt, bananas, maple syrup and vanilla extract until smooth.
4. Stir in the oats, baking soda and cinnamon until combined.
5. Finally, stir in the flour until just combined and fold in the cacao nibs (and broken nuts).
6. Pour the mixture into a baking tin and bake until a toothpick or knife inserted into the centre comes out clean. The time depends on the dimensions of your pan, roughly 25 minutes.
7. Remove from the oven and leave to cool on a cooling rack.
8. This banana bread is best served warm, so there's no need to hang around!

Even if the bread has cooled fully some time later, a quick blast in the microwave, followed up with a teaspoon of light butter, and you'll be in all kinds of heaven!

COGNITION – WHAT IS IT? HOW AND WHY DOES FASTING IMPROVE IT?

"The mental action or process of acquiring knowledge and understanding through thought, experience, and the senses.". To put it simply, cognition is your brainpower! Many might assume that in the absence of incoming food, your brain would fall limp, but it's actually quite the opposite, and the research behind this fact is extensive.

Before we delve into fasting's effect on the brain, let's step back once again to the evolutionary perspective. Max Lugavere, author of 'Genius Foods', summarises this point perfectly, "When we are fasted, our brains are actually primed to be at their most clever. As hunter-gatherers, we wouldn't have made it very far as a species if we became less intelligent when food ceased to be readily available.". Still not convinced? Then allow me to bring you forward to the present day, to what the research has to say....

Fasting can be seen as a healthy type of stress for the brain, just like exercise. Under good stress, your brain induces a stress response, producing a number of molecules. These include orexin-A and norepinephrine, the effect of these being a heightened sense of awareness, sharpened senses, and increased focus and memory.[17][18] Fasting also increases levels of ketone bodies, including beta-hydroxybutyrate (BHB), which have the capacity to supply up to 75% of the brain's energy needs.[19] BHB acts as a potent fuel source for the brain when glucose levels run low, as it can easily cross the blood-brain barrier.

A common misconception is that your brain needs 130g of carbohydrates to function; however, the stress response induced, along with the production of ketone bodies, is just one of the reasons that this is not this case. As we also know from Angus Barbieri, after 380 days of fasting, his blood glucose remained constant since the liver is capable of producing glucose from glycerol, which is produced from the breakdown of stored fat, and so the brain will be supplied with carbohydrates without them even being consumed!

Now the kicker. Stressful stimuli, like fasting and exercises, are like challenges for your brain, and such challenges increase the level of certain neurotrophic factors, such as BDNF. In basic terms, BDNF helps protect your brain cells, aids in producing new brain cells and facilitates the neurons in your brain wiring together, which is what learning is.[20] Not only does BDNF boost 'brainpower' and memory, but it's also associated with improved mood and increased productivity.

So, what is the effect of fasting on BDNF levels? A 2% increase? A 5% increase? A study was performed to find out the effect of fasting during Ramadan on BDNF levels, and after just 14 days, participants showed a 25% increase in BDNF, an already significant jump, but it didn't stop there. The full 29 days through the trial, participants displayed a 47% increase in BDNF! The results of this study clearly display the positive correlation between fasting and BDNF, which is especially staggering given the short time span of the procedure.[21]

Like all the best things in life, there is no wide-open path to improved cognition. Standing before this sought-after benefit is a cloud, a cloud of hunger, irritability and distraction, all of which can be combated through a period of adaptation. So, in the beginning, be sure not to see them as a red flag! It's also important to note that the factors affecting these hurdles span far beyond fasting, and it's completely natural to have them come and go from time to time.

"I fast for greater physical and mental efficiency."
– Plato

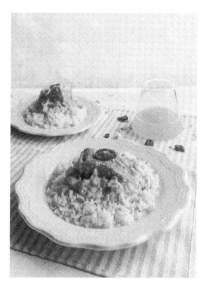

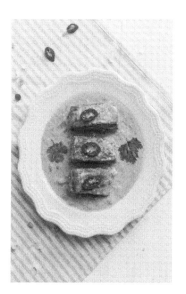

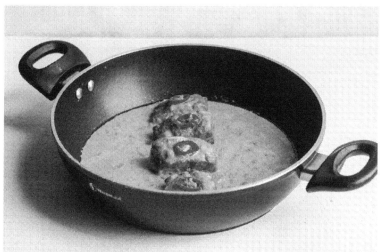

31

COCONUT SALMON WITH SPRING ONION RICE – SERVES 4

Ingredients:

2 tsps ground cumin

2 tsps chilli powder

1 tsp turmeric

2 tbsps white wine vinegar (alternative: lemon juice or apple cider vinegar)

A pinch of salt and pepper

4 salmon fillets (alternative: chickpeas)

250g basmati rice

750ml water

1 tsp cumin seeds

5-6 cardamom pods

1 generous tsp coconut oil

1 onion chopped

2 fresh chillies or a good pinch of chilli flakes (reduce for less heat)

2 garlic cloves

A thumb of slice ginger

1 tsp ground coriander

1 can of coconut milk

2 chopped spring onions

A pinch of fresh coriander

Method:

1. In a small bowl, mix the first teaspoon of ground cumin, along with the chilli powder, turmeric, vinegar, salt and pepper to make a paste.
2. Rub the paste over the salmon fillets and leave to marinate for 10-15 minutes – get the rest of your ingredients ready whilst it sits!
3. In a large deep sided frying pan, heat coconut oil on a medium-high heat and fry onion, chillies, ginger and garlic for 5 minutes.
4. Add the remaining teaspoon of ground cumin, along with ground coriander and coconut milk, lower the heat and simmer for 5-10 minutes.
5. Add the salmon fillets to the pan, coating them with the coconut sauce. Cover and cook for 15 minutes, or until the fish is tender.
6. Add rice, water, cumin seeds and cardamom pods to a saucepan and bring to the boil before reducing to a gentle simmer for 10 minutes whilst the salmon cooks – keep an eye on the rice and add a splash of water if it should need it throughout the cooking.
7. Mix the chopped spring onions through the rice and garnish the salmon with fresh coriander.
8. Serve the rice and salmon side by side, and don't forget a serving spoon for all that sauce!

HUNGER AND HOW TO KEEP A LID ON IT

The biggest roadblock faced when trying to control what we eat is hunger. The feeling that diverts your attention towards feeding yourself. When poorly managed, hunger consumes a lot of mental strain; this can be especially true when starting out with fasting. So, how can we combat hunger? First, we must understand what this feeling is and how it comes about.

What Causes Hunger?

Our present perception of hunger is widely oversimplified; it's not just a case of the less you eat, the hungrier you get. Hunger works in a cyclical nature, dictated by your usual eating habits. When you approach one of your 'usual' mealtimes, you receive a spike in a hormone called ghrelin, and you get hungry. What you may not know is that once you surpass the window you usually eat in, even if you don't eat, ghrelin reduces and your hunger goes away until your next expected mealtime.

As we all know, the primary way to combat hunger is by consuming food, which leads to feeling satiated (full). Leptin is the primary satiety hormone; it's in charge of how full you feel. Leptin levels can differ, depending on the composition of your meals, both size and macronutrient levels. So, in basic terms, that's it, hunger is a balance between leptin and ghrelin, and the great news is that there are many factors that influence the levels of these hormones, which is what we will aim to manipulate.

Steps to Tackle Hunger

Now first up, fasting alone can go a long way in building a great relationship with hunger. Remember what I said back in 'Extended Fasting'? "In fact, extended periods of fasting decrease your overall levels of ghrelin, which control your hunger signals. So, over time, you actually get less and less hungry, providing you don't eat!".[23] Hunger is also a completely natural process and one that you should not aim to avoid entirely. However, it can be a bit of a nuisance at times, especially when you're switching to a new eating pattern. Hence why I've put together some practical steps to undertake if hunger ever gets out of control.

1 - Hydration

The first place you should turn when you feel hungry is to water. Dehydration can provide the same discomfort as hunger, so it can easily fly under the radar. And so, my first suggestion would be to drink a sufficient amount of water and wait 10-15 minutes. If your discomfort hasn't passed, continue to examine your feelings.

2 - Cravings

There are a number of scenarios you might find yourself in that lead you to believe you're hungry, when you're actually just craving. Recognising these situations mean that when they do arise, you're aware that they may be the cause of what seems to be hunger. Are you bored? Did you just experience an acutely stressful situation? Are you tired? If you've just broken your fast, are you letting the floodgates open? More on this point overleaf.

Specific cravings can also arise as your body's way of telling you that you're not satisfying its need for a certain nutrient. Low carbohydrate diets can lead to sugar cravings. Restricting your salt intake too much can lead you to crave salty (often fast) foods. A quick way to recognise this is to ask yourself, "In this moment, could I eat anything?", say a plain ham sandwich or a pickle (choose anything that works for you). If yes, you may well just be hungry. If not, consider that maybe your body is in need of a certain nutrient.

How to minimise or move past cravings? Firstly, try to adjust your diet, based on the specific things you crave to ensure you're giving your body what it needs. Alternatively, as I like to say, plug them. My personal approach to cravings is like a game of whack-a-mole. Once they start to arise, I whack them back down like a mole, satisfying them as soon as possible. The longer cravings linger, the harder you're going to have to hit them to alleviate them.

Letting the Flood Gates Open as Soon as You're in Your Feeding Window

The reward centres in your brain may switch to food as a reward for abstaining from it, in the form of indulgence – almost like 'feeding time'. This can be especially the case for longer periods of fasting. My first suggestion to tame this would be to follow the same process as mentioned for hunger and cravings. Alternatively, the breathing technique below may help to 'ride the wave' of hunger. Seeing this as a wave that will go as quickly as it came also provides a lot of psychological ease. Finally, you could satisfy this want for consumption with something that isn't going to set you back, something light but still satisfying - see my craving crusher below.

Simple 4:7:8 Breathing Technique

1. Find a comfortable position whether that be seated, standing or lying down – maintain an upright posture.
2. Breathe in for a count of four.
3. Hold the breath for a count of seven.
4. Breathe out for a count of eight.
5. Repeat this cycle four times.

A Craving Crusher for On-the-go

An all-time craving and sweet tooth crusher of mine when dieting is a flat white with almond milk and two squares of Godiva's 90% dark chocolate. Specific, I know, and also very simplistic. Easy to have on the go, and something about it just hits the spot for me! I even have a specific way of having it that makes it so great, but I could never tell you that – Hint: Warm coffee melts chocolate.

3 - Hunger

Maybe what you're feeling is hunger, so what now? Like I introduced previously, hunger is a balance between leptin and ghrelin, both of which can be kept in check. Below are a number of ways you can do this; hence, managing the feelings they provide.

Ghrelin - Feel Less Hungry

Your body is extremely well-designed to adapt to changing circadian rhythms; light (jet lag), temperature, eating pattern... Due to the cyclical nature of ghrelin, over time, you can alter what part of the day you feel hungry, with mealtimes that you dictate. Here, it really is as simple as following a new eating schedule and allowing your body time to adapt! In the process of adapting, many will see the discomfort as a red flag, but it's a necessary process. Keep in mind that during this phase, you will find the periods where you usually eat especially difficult.

Other steps that can be taken to manage ghrelin include getting good quality sleep and managing your method of caloric restriction, something you'll see at play in the following chapter. Implementing diet breaks and refeeds can also be a great asset if you're in a period of weight loss.

Leptin - Feel More Full

Fasting alone can go a long way in managing leptin through insulin. To keep it simple, insulin blocks leptin, and fasting reduces insulin. You can further reduce insulin, or spikes in insulin, by manipulating carbohydrate consumption. Reducing carbs, maybe just for a period of the day, or slowly introducing them throughout the day, can be a great way to keep hunger at bay. Having said this, especially given the already shortened window to eat, if you function better or prefer a higher carbohydrate diet, then this point may add needless complexity to the process!

So, as we know, leptin is in-charge of making you feel satiated (full). Eating more satiating foods can, therefore, keep leptin levels in check. Foods that are high in protein and fibre are highly satiating, so be sure to integrate them into your meals throughout the day. Protein also has a high 'thermic effect', which means it requires more energy to digest. Up to 30% of the calories from protein you consume are used to break it down, so if you eat 100 calories of protein, only 70 calories are actually usable! Fats also provide a great deal of satiation; however, this must be balanced with the higher calorie content they provide.

A great way to break your fast may be tuna, eggs, avocado, and olive oil, providing a lasting feeling of fullness, introducing carbohydrates later as the day goes on.

Next, foods that are high in volume and low in energy density are a great way to almost 'cheat' hunger. Here, you needn't look far beyond vegetables, especially leafy greens. To put this idea of energy density into context: Half a kilo of kale has a mere 245 calories; I'm not sure I can even picture how much kale that is, never mind eating it. Half a kilo of peanuts? 2,835. Now let me be clear, all foods have a place in any diet, and there should be no 'bad' foods. However, if you're struggling to manage hunger, consider the ratio of volume: calories, and tip the scales either way when you feel you can or want to.

Examples of high volume, low-calorie foods are: High fibre fruit, vegetables and big leafy salads. Low-fat Greek yogurt, popcorn and even oats when prepared correctly are all super high in volume for their calorie content – you can prepare the oats by ensuring you add lots of water and cooking them for slightly longer! And a final go-to from my back pocket, egg white frittatas! Another really easy low-calorie option; you can check out my recipe for these.

But first, one last reminder! You can always resort to taking a few deep breaths. This sounds cliché, but there's method behind the madness. There is a huge psychological influence on hunger; likewise, stress can be a major cause. If your hunger ever gets out of control, stop, take a few deep breaths, or practice the breathing exercise listed. Continue using the points discussed to pinpoint why it could be happening and whether or not there's something that can be done about it. Or, just ride the wave while it passes!

> *"Hunger is the first element of self-discipline. If you can*
> *control what you eat and drink, you can control everything else"*
> *– Dr. Umar Faruq Abd-Allah*

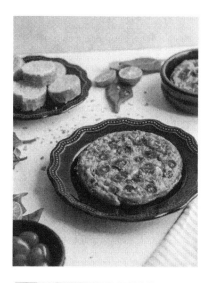
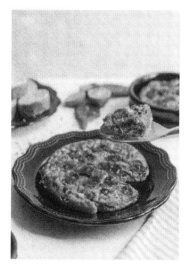
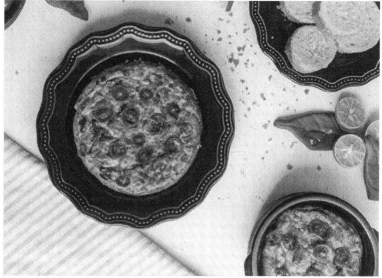

BOMBAY EGG WHITE FRITTATA – SERVES 1

Ingredients:

4 eggs or 2 eggs and 4 egg whites
75ml almond milk
50g or ½ a green pepper
100g or 1 medium red onion
80g or 1 medium tomato
A handful of spinach
1 tsp of chilli flakes, cumin seeds, turmeric and garam masala
Squeeze of lemon or lime juice
(Add any other vegetables)

Method:

1. Preheat your oven to 180°C degrees.
2. Beat the eggs (and egg whites), almond milk, turmeric and garam masala to make the egg mixture.
3. In a skillet or pan suitable for the oven, fry peppers, red onion, tomatoes, spinach, chilli flakes and cumin seeds with a squeeze of lemon or lime juice (you can use a low-calorie oil spray, but not using oil will reduce the calories).
4. Once fried, add the egg mixture and cook 3 minutes or so before adding the pan to the oven to cook for 15-20 minutes - if pan has a handle, leave the oven door open.
5. Serve the frittata, running a spatula around the edge to keep it whole, and enjoy!

AN EFFECTIVE WEIGHT LOSS STRATEGY THAT PROTECTS YOUR METABOLISM

The Role of Insulin

Insulin, we've all heard of it, but what does it really do? Insulin is a hormone that allows your body to convert the food you're consuming into energy, ready to be used or stored for later as either glycogen or fat. This means it plays a major role in maintaining stable blood glucose levels. High levels of insulin have been linked to obesity, heart disease and cancer. It also stops leptin (the satiety hormone in-charge of making you feel full) from working and blocks your ability to use stored fat, which I discuss below. Keeping your insulin levels regulated is vital for good health and weight management, and intermittent fasting alone has been found to effectively reduce insulin levels. It also increases insulin sensitivity; this allows the cells in your body to use blood glucose more effectively, a major reason why fasting is met with stable energy levels.[24]

When you eat, insulin rises, and your body is in 'storing mode'. When you don't eat, insulin falls, and your body moves into 'burning mode'. If insulin levels are high, in order to tap into fat stores, your glycogen stores have to be sufficiently low, the freezer is padlocked until the fridge is sufficiently empty; this is calorie restriction. However, if your insulin levels are low, glycogen levels do not have to be low for you to tap into this stored fat. In this case, the padlock is off the freezer, even before the fridge is empty, and this can be done by fasting.

Metabolism and Hunger

Metabolism simply describes all of the chemical reactions in your body that keep you alive. We use the basal metabolic rate (BMR) as a measure of how many calories your body requires to function at rest. So, how does fasting affect your metabolism when compared with calorie restriction? This was the question Catenacci and colleagues had when they set out to pit the two against one another in 2016. Over the course of an 8 week study, the team compared intermittent fasting with regular calorie constriction, and there is one major finding I'd like to highlight; the calorie restriction group saw a significant reduction in BMR, whilst the fasting group did not.[12]

Now, what we also know is that regular calorie restriction increases the levels of ghrelin, the hunger hormone. So, looking at the overall picture, your body is making you function on fewer calories, whilst increasing hunger in a bid to make you eat more calories. Reducing metabolism and increasing hunger is your body's attempt to get you back to your previous weight. In order to continue losing weight, you must continue to restrict your calories, and with each incremental restriction, your metabolism falls further, and hunger levels climb. This can be seen in the practical examples overleaf.

If we take a look at fasting on a larger scale, a 3-day fast was also found to increase BMR by roughly 12% during the 3-day period.[18] Why does this happen? Once again, due to the cavalry of counter-regulatory hormones that help you maintain muscle, whose job is to keep you functioning optimally in the absence of food.

Practical Examples

The following practical examples show two possible methods for weight loss. The first is normal calorie restriction; the second is the same calorie restriction using a fasting protocol. Using these two cases, I also weigh in on the flaws of the basic 'calories in vs. calories out' idea. There is much debate on this subject, but my opinion is that human physiology is complex, and although calories are a great metric to track your energy consumption, they're extremely simplistic. They do not consider factors such as the hormonal responses to what you consume, nor the effect your consumption can have on your metabolism. These examples tell the story better than I can... in both cases, we assume a maintenance calorie intake of 2,200.

Example 1 - Regular Calorie Restriction:

You reduce your calorie intake to say, 1,800 calories, insulin coming and going throughout the day as you eat, how much depending on the composition of your meals. During the day, you cannot effectively use stored fat as an energy source as insulin is present, so, over time, your body responds by reducing metabolism to 1,800 calories, as this is the energy it has available to use. Calories in still equal calories out, no laws of thermodynamics broken, simply your body reducing its energy expenditure to match the energy it has at its disposal. (This is not exact and throughout this process, yes, you will lose some weight)

Over time, you are left with a new base metabolism, tending towards 1,800 calories. In order to continue losing weight, you must further restrict your calories, to say 1,600 calories, until your metabolism follows suit, down to 1,600. This cycle continues, and yes, you may very well achieve your weight loss goal, but where is your metabolism left? Lower than you'd probably like. The process of your metabolism falling will be seen as a reduction in felt energy and a general slowing down of the body. All the while, hunger is increasing.

Example 2 – Calorie Restriction on a Fasting Protocol:

So, how is fasting any different? You reduce your calories on a fasting protocol, again to 1,800, and since insulin is sufficiently low for a large period of the day, you are better able to use stored fat for energy, hence why your metabolism can maintain much closer to 2,200. This is supported by the research stated above. Some of the remaining 400 calories of energy you need will have been accessed through stored fat (example figures, not exact); hence, you lose weight, and your metabolism stays better intact. As you continue to lose weight, you are still energetic, both for reasons discussed at length in the 'Energy' chapter and since your metabolism is stable. What's more! As we know from the previous chapter, hunger and cravings are also kept at bay.

Please note, these examples are very simplistic for explanation purposes. Any eating plan that restricts your calories will eventually decrease your metabolism over an extended period of time; however, fasting can slow this reduction, for the reasons discussed above. Extended periods of caloric restriction, fasting or otherwise, can also lead to increased hunger. Again, here, fasting can simply mitigate this increase.

Final Thoughts on Weight Loss

Weight loss may rule the captions of Instagram posts and YouTube videos, with quick fixes, tips and tricks around every corner, but there are a few fundamentals that are often skipped over. Firstly, weight loss should not come at the cost of quality of life. The likelihood is, if it does encroach too far on quality of life, it won't be sustainable anyway. This doesn't mean weight loss won't be difficult, just not detrimental.

Enter a phase of weight loss having sustained a stable weight for some time. Your body has energy demands, and if you don't supply them, it will reduce its ability to function to match what you give it. Chronic calorie restriction manifests itself in all sorts of ways, from low mood and anxiety, to reduced thyroid function, to extreme hunger and food focus. Ensure you have sustained periods of sufficient eating, which will also make weight loss a whole lot easier when you do come to it.

We are all made of different genetic make-up, we all distribute weight on our body differently, we all gain and lose weight at different rates. Subsequently, how we should each treat our body will be different. Let the information you read guide you, collecting all the tools in the armoury that you might need, to then be your own best expert and apply them to suit your biological individuality. And no matter what you read online, there is far more to the picture than calories.

"Every human being is the author of his
own health or disease"
– Buddha

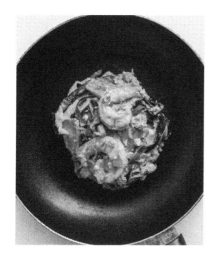

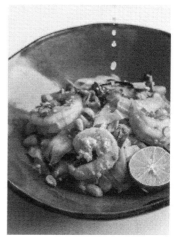

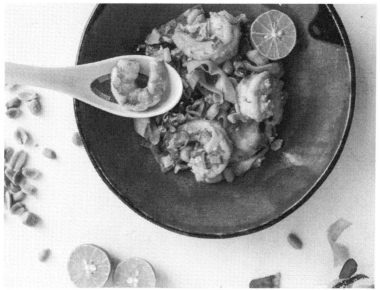

LOW CARB PRAWN PAD THAI – SERVES 1

Ingredients:

1 large courgette
3 carrots (skin peeled off)
Low calorie spray or olive oil
100ml water
1 garlic clove
1 serving prawns, uncooked – grey (alternative: precooked prawns or fried tofu)
1 egg
2 tbsps lemon juice (a replacement for tamarind that I prefer)
2 tbsps fish sauce
1 tsp of sriracha, or a pinch of dried or fresh chilli.
1 tsp honey
1 flat tbsp crunchy peanut butter or crushed peanuts
A crack of salt and pepper
1 handful beansprouts
A pinch of coriander
A thumb of sliced spring onion
¼ lime wedge

Method:

1. If you have a spiraliser, spiralise the courgette and carrots. Otherwise, take a peeler and peel, peel, peel away to make ribbons. If the final parts are a pain to peel, thinly slice (no waste!).
2. Line a wok or pan with low calorie oil spray or add a splash of olive oil and wipe the olive oil around the surface with a napkin to coat the wok.
3. Add garlic and fry for 1 minute before adding carrot and courgette and water, along with lemon juice, fish sauce, honey, peanut butter, salt and pepper. Cover to steam for 10 minutes.
4. Add the prawns and continue cooking for 5 minutes.
5. Push the contents of the wok to one side (or to the edges to make a space in the centre) and crack in the egg, break and scramble as you would scrambled eggs.
6. Once eggs are scrambled, add bean sprouts and combine all contents of the pan.
7. Taste and add additional sriracha (for heat), honey (for sweetness) or peanut butter (for nuttiness).
8. Garnish with coriander and spring onion, and serve with soy sauce (instead of adding salt!) and a lime wedge on the side to add to taste.

FASTING FOR GUT HEALTH

We are just starting to scratch the surface to understand the role and effects our gut health and microbiome have on our overall wellbeing. If I hadn't suddenly faced gut issues myself, I'm not convinced I would have been able to gain the knowledge on the subject that I have up to this point. To give a brief outline, the gut is the group of organs that make up the digestive system. Residing within this group of organs is a vast ecosystem of microbes, including bacteria, fungi and viruses. These microbes "contribute metabolic functions, protect against pathogens, educate the immune system, and, through these basic functions, affect, directly or indirectly, most of our physiologic functions.".[25] The state of your gut microbiome will also affect both how you digest different foods and also how hungry or full you feel![26]

You can picture managing your gut health like tending to a garden. There will always be "good" and "bad" microbes, and maintaining a balanced variety of these microbes is the goal of maintaining a healthy, happy gut. Much like a garden, your gut health cannot be overhauled overnight. A bottle of kefir here and there, nor a kombucha once a month won't have nearly the impact of a balanced diet, or, based on lots of promising research, fasting! A 2016 paper by Fetissov states, "strong experimental evidence suggests that not only diet but also feeding schedules are important determinants for microbiota composition and function.".[26]

Intermittent fasting can improve the diversity of the microbes in the gut, also helping to fend off those that are less wanted. A 2018 study performed on individuals with multiple sclerosis found that intermittent fasting led to an increased gut bacteria richness and enrichment of the Lactobacillaceae, Bacteroidaceae, and Prevotellaceae families.[14] Noting especially here that Lactobacillus is heavily supported for its positive effects on gut health. Another 2015 study found an increase in the species 'Akkermansia' as a result of intermittent fasting, which has been shown to reduce fat mass gain and improve gut barrier function and glucose metabolism.[27]

Circadian Rhythm

The circadian rhythm is the process that regulates the sleep-wake cycle; it may surprise you to know that certain microbes in the gut also have a circadian rhythm! This means that gut microbes can ramp up when food is expected, during the day, and wind down as the day comes to a close at night. Ensuring that you only eat when your body is primed to metabolise food can improve insulin sensitivity, lower insulin levels and also decrease appetite.[27] Not to mention keeping the bugs in your gut happy! Research finds that the disruption of the microbiome circadian rhythm is associated with metabolic disease.[26]

The Gut Wall

The intestinal wall within our gut, or epithelium, plays an important role in absorbing nutrients from the food that you consume. If the structure of this wall becomes compromised, this can lead to "leaky gut", or increased intestinal permeability, where unwanted bacteria and toxins can seep through the wall of the gut. This can, in turn, lead to an inflammatory response, skin irritation, bloating, and an inability to absorb nutrients effectively. Fasting can provide the necessary rest for the gut epithelium to heal or help to avoid this issue in the first place. Speaking from personal experience, I have suffered from leaky gut due to an extended course of misprescribed antibiotics, and found a noticeable improvement in symptoms from periods of gut rest through fasting. Finally, be sure to practice caution with coffee on an empty stomach, for the sake of your gut wall! I'll discuss this in a little more detail in an upcoming chapter.

There is No Replacement for Diet

Whilst the current research looks favourably on intermittent fasting for gut health; there is no replacement for a balanced diet that's supportive of your gut health needs. "Eating habits are the main significant determinants of the microbial multiplicity of the gut, and dietary components influence both microbial populations and their metabolic activities from the early stages of life."[28] Limiting refined sugar and artificial sweeteners and consuming regular fermented foods like kefir, kombucha and sauerkraut can support further support digestive health. A good probiotic and prebiotics, including onions, garlic, leeks and green bananas, can balance the level of "good" and "bad" bacteria, with prebiotics feeding the good. Dietary fibre, zinc and l-glutamine supplementation can retain the integrity of the gut wall, also reducing gut inflammation.[29][30]

A final mention for bone broth can also be made. Besides containing a host of vitamins, minerals and collagen, it contains high levels of anti-inflammatory amino acids that can help to heal the intestinal wall and aid those with digestive issues, such as IBS.[30][31] You'll find my go-to bone broth recipe at the end of this chapter, which I used to consume every day when I had gut problems – it's a bit of a throw it together based on what I usually had available! I start from a whole chicken and show you how to make the broth itself and a killer noodle soup using one serving of the broth!

Bonus tip: Dilute up to 2 tablespoons of apple cider vinegar with half a small can or bottle of kombucha with some still or sparkling water. This spreads kombucha (which is often expensive) over 2 servings and can make a tasty sparkling drink.

"Fasting gives your body time to heal itself. It relieves nervousness and tension and gives your digestive system a rest."
– Jentezen Franklin

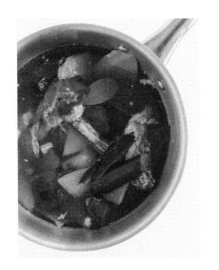
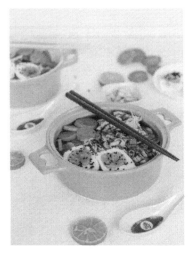
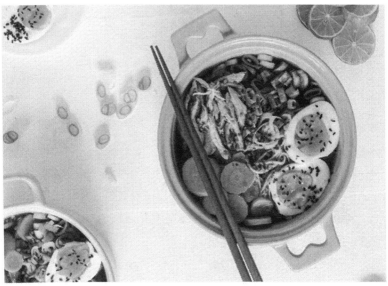

BONE BROTH AND KILLER NOODLE SOUP

The recipe assumes your pot to be a generic large saucepan, producing roughly 4/5 servings.

Ingredients:

1 whole chicken
1 tbsp turmeric
Crack of salt and pepper
Selection of vegetables for the noodle soup. Go ahead and grab whatever is at your disposal! Leeks, cabbage, onions, beansprouts, peppers, whatever takes your pick.
Water (sufficient to fill your chosen pot 2 cm from the top)
8 tbsp apple cider vinegar (the acidity breaks down the collagen, making it more available) – roughly 2 tablespoons per serving. (alternative: lemon juice)

For My Go-To Interpretation:

At this point, you can either get creative and/or use up any scraps, leftovers or herbs gone dry that are lying around.

1 tbsp coconut oil – having numerous health and digestive benefits
1 tbsp lemon juice
A generous helping of soy sauce or coconut aminos
A generous thumb of sliced ginger - skin and all if you like
2-3 cloves of crushed/sliced garlic
1 stick of lemon grass, or a tbsp of puree
6 or so bay leaves
1 tbsp turmeric

Dried or crushed chilli to preference - a few small dried chilli or a tbsp of flakes. I like the heat!

5 or so cloves (optional - strong flavour, but great for digestion)

1 tbsp fennel seeds - again, great for digestion

A generous crack of black pepper – to activate the curcumin in the turmeric, a potent anti-inflammatory and antioxidant

Salt to taste - be careful, the soy sauce brings salt to the table too!

Method:

1. Marinate the chicken in olive oil, turmeric, salt and black pepper and cook in a pre-heated oven at 190°C for 1 hour 30 minutes, simple.

2. With 30 minutes left until cooked, remove your chicken and add your choice of vegetables to the flavour filled roasting dish, either around or under the chicken, putting it back in the oven for the remaining 30 minutes.

3. Carve the chicken, keeping the meat and vegetables aside, and place all that remains in your chosen saucepan.

4. Optional but recommended step: Instead of adding the chicken carcass to the pot, place it back into the oven until it has a dark caramel colour before adding it to the pot. This starts the break down process and adds an unbeaten depth of flavour.

5. Fill the saucepan with water, leaving roughly 2cm of room at the top.

6. Add all of your additional ingredients, bring to the boil and then reduce the heat to a very gentle simmer.

7. Cover your saucepan and leave to simmer for up to 12 hours, yes you heard right, 12 hours - I would suggest a minimum of 6 hours. The longer you leave your broth, the better. I would recommend leaving it from morning to night, so you can keep an eye on it. Be

sure not to leave the heat too high, the aim is to reduce the liquid by roughly half. You may need to top the saucepan up throughout cooking to achieve this if the minimum heat you have is still too high. Please do not let the liquid to boil away, allowing the pan to burn!

8. Once the broth has finished simmering, pass the liquid from the saucepan through a sieve or strainer into a bowl or glassware of your choice.

9. Leave to cool, do not add the broth straight to the fridge!

10. Once cooled, the broth can be added to the fridge and kept fresh for a handful of days. You can also freeze it for later use. Note, at this point, the broth may turn into a jelly-like consistency, this is perfectly normal!

How to serve:

11. Serve and enjoy the broth hot as a stand-alone by adding a few tablespoons into a mug with boiling water, or incorporate into a dish of your choice, like a noodle soup! Alternatively, use the chicken and vegetables for a different dish.

12. For a killer noodle soup, add around $\frac{1}{4}$ of your broth per serving to a saucepan topped with water – the amount of water varies largely on the number of servings, serving bowl size and saucepan size; trust your intuition here.

13. Once boiling, add the chicken, flavour filled veggies and your choice of noodles.

14. Cover and leave until the noodles are cooked, rest to thicken up and serve! You can also top with a runny egg!

STRESS - THE GOOD
AND THE BAD

Many healthy lifestyle choices can cause an abundance of stress if made to be too restrictive, followed too rigidly, or practiced too often. So much so that any potential benefits are far outweighed. The right kind of stress, in moderation, isn't a bad thing. In fact, it's a good thing! A healthy dose of stress can be highly beneficial to us. Keeping this dose to a healthy limit, however, is something to be wary of, as once this spills over, it can start to cause us all kinds of issues, including hormone imbalances and inflammation.

Deciding what to eat and when to eat it can be very mentally taxing. If you find that keeping careful track of what you eat can become a little too much, creating a period of the day where the choice is removed, fasting, followed by a period where you can be relaxed about food, can make this equation much simpler. On the other hand, if the mental distraction of not eating entirely detracts from a given period of the day, fasting during this period may not be for you.

If you're sat by the TV, and everyone's tucking into their favourite snacks around you, but you're outside the time you've chosen to eat, sitting and watching them while your mind is closer to the fridge than it is on enjoying yourself is clearly not the right approach. In that moment, it may just be "healthier" for you to tuck into whatever it is you crave, so you can put your mind to rest and relax, rather than stewing over the situation you find yourself in.

On the flip side, in this situation, you might not actually want anything, you may be aware that you've indulged a lot recently, or it just wouldn't be worth it anyway, so you don't have to deviate. It's a surprisingly fine line between showing constraint and chaining yourself down; that's why it's so important to become your own personal expert on what you need to find that sustainable balance.

Stressful stimulus comes in many forms in the modern world, and these must be managed collectively. Fasting itself comes with its own stress response, as seen by a rise in cortisol, the primary stress hormone.[22] For this reason, an individual can 'over-fast', especially if in conjunction with other stressors. Again, you must be your own personal expert here, as everyone encounters a different amount of stress and also tolerates this stress differently. Be sure to check in with yourself and your stress levels regularly, especially if you are prone to anxiety. But wait! Be sure not to overanalyse where this stress is coming from; it's very easy to build false associations with what's causing something like stress. And a bonus tip! Coffee also increases cortisol, so a fasted period fuelled with coffee may be a little on the stressful side! Try switching to green tea once and a while, which contains the calming amino acid l-theanine.

When it comes to living a healthy lifestyle, there comes a point at which pursuing this lifestyle comes at the cost of the stress provided by the process. Now, this may seem trivial, "surely this acute stress is far outweighed by all these wonderful benefits". Whilst it may seem this way, stressful situations accumulate, and the mind is also a powerful thing. So, be sure to continually check in with yourself and weigh up whether the stress provided by this seamlessly "healthy" lifestyle choice actually allows it to continue serving you. Oh yeah! And if you are ever feeling stressed and need to take your mind off things, why not try my guilt-free "Breakfast or Dessert Pizza" recipe!

> *"The paths to paradise are many, fasting is one of them."*
> *– Mufti Menk*

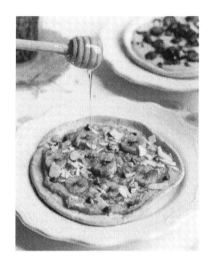

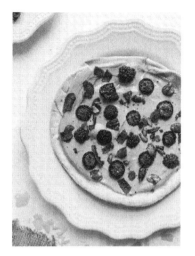

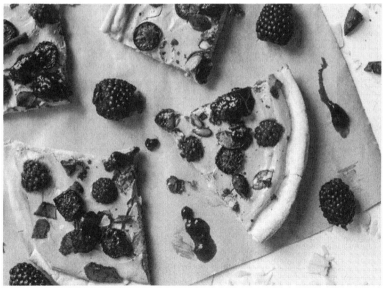

BREAKFAST DESSERT PIZZA...
NOT ONE TO MISS! – SERVES 2

Ingredients:

2 wraps of choice
3 tbsps low fat yogurt
1 tsp cocoa powder
Alternative peanut butter base: 2 tbsps powdered peanut butter with 2 tbsps of water.

Toppings:

Anything you want really!

1 banana
2 handfuls berries (I used frozen raspberries and blueberries)
2 handfuls of granola
For peanut butter base, dark chocolate buttons work great!

Remove any toppings to your preference or throw on something completely different!

Method:

1. Preheat your oven to 180°C.
2. For a cocoa base, combine low fat yogurt with cocoa powder. For alternative peanut butter base, combine powdered peanut butter with water.
3. Cover your wrap of choice with your chosen base!
4. Add toppings. For the cocoa base, I used banana, frozen blueberries and raspberries, and a sprinkle of granola. For the nut butter base, I used banana, dark chocolate buttons and frozen raspberries.
5. Cook the pizza in the oven until the edges of the wrap start to brown; this should take around 5 minutes.
6. Serve and enjoy!

THE FASTED LIFESTYLE

Throughout this book, I've referred to intermittent fasting as a 'lifestyle', as opposed to a 'diet'. I truly do believe intermittent fasting to be about much more than the food you eat, when you eat it, and how it affects your health. It touches all corners of your life, from productivity to willpower, structure to financials, all playing a key role in what I call 'The Fasted Lifestyle'. I can say for certain that I would have achieved a fraction of what I have now without the lifestyle that intermittent fasting provides. The points mentioned here only scratch the surface, I'm sure of it. They are, however, the ones that stuck out to me through my personal experience. If I hadn't busted one final myth already, "Intermittent fasting is crazy", then here goes my final say...

Willpower and Decision

Willpower is like a muscle; the more you work it, the more fatigued it gets. It also has a limit to how far it can be stretched before you concede. The number of decisions that revolve around food and drink are surprisingly large, especially in a modern world with so much choice. When you fast, you take these decisions and all of their choices off the table entirely, at least for a portion of the day. That vital willpower that only stretches so far can now be spent elsewhere on other decisions of the day.

Time & Productivity

I've paired these two points together, as they go hand in hand. The time taken to cook, eat, clean and digest food cannot be underestimated. How many times have you rushed to get out of the door because you needed to get your breakfast down? Leaving a complete mess in your wake. The morning has become the most productive time of day for me. Having adapted to the process, you have stable energy, with no crash from digesting a meal, all with your full attention devoted to what you need to do. With the morning period often dictating how the rest of your day will go, I've found this to be hugely beneficial.

Save Money

Now off the bat, I don't want you to get the wrong end of the stick; my point is not, restricting yourself leads you to spend less. The point I am making is that accumulating small purchases can really add up, and once again, removing the choice when it comes to food purchases can quite seamlessly reduce the number of purchases you make. By generally consuming fewer meals during the day, you limit the need to buy meals out, with it also being much easier to prepare and carry food. Note, this isn't the case for everyone's situation! But in many cases, especially if you're in another country, or you're away from home, it can really cut things down.

Structure

Although I often recommend not getting too caught up in the start and finish times that you eat, having a regimented eating schedule that you can carry across any time zone can add a great deal of structure to your day. I also find that having a line between fasting and eating allows you to allocate your time accordingly, focusing on the tasks that require the most attention in the morning, whilst you have it, introducing food as the day goes on... maybe finishing the day back at home with sufficient time to enjoy the process of cooking and eating. With eating playing a huge role in the body's circadian rhythm, having this structure to your eating can also help to regulate your sleep-wake cycle.

Simplify Your Life

Whilst many 'diets' add complications and constraints to your life, intermittent fasting may simplify it. Having a period of the day where you're free from food, before a period where you can be at ease with what you're eating, may be extremely beneficial to some. You're just fasting, then you're eating. Whilst I have nothing against tracking calories and do myself from time to time, I feel that monitoring everything you consume just isn't a sustainable or particularly free way to live. Intermittent fasting might just be the key to the constraints for you on that front.

Can Be Incorporated Under Most Circumstances

Whether your choice of eating is vegan, vegetarian, pescatarian, low carb, high carb, ketogenic, you name it; it can be done in accordance with fasting. Allergic to peanuts, lactose intolerant, coeliac… it can be done in accordance with fasting. Too busy, not enough money… you get the idea. In most circumstances, intermittent fasting can be practiced regardless of the other lifestyle choices you make, which is extremely valuable. Even as your day-to-day life changes, say, going aboard, intermittent fasting can be carried along with you.

"The discipline of fasting breaks you out
of the worlds routine."
– Jentezen Franklin

Myths That Just Got Busted

Myth 1: Fasting causes you to burn muscle

Myth 2: You have no energy without consuming food, your brain and body need 130g of carbohydrates to function

Myth 3: Fasting makes your brain fall limp

Myth 4: The less you eat, the hungrier you get

Myth 5: Fasting slows your metabolism, eating every 2-hours keeps your metabolism going

Myth 6: Fasting starves all the bacteria in your gut

Myth 7: Intermittent fasting is crazy

THE FASTED PERIO

THE

FAST

SPEC

FASTI

MODERN DAY FASTING

ADVANCED TECHNIQUES

GETTING STARTED

What you can and can't consu
many will tell you different
what you're trying to a
sacrifice. When it co
point in greater
to what you'
what ca
that

ɪe during a fast is an open verdict, and
y. In my opinion, it really comes down to
chieve and what you're realistically willing to
mes to what you're trying to achieve, I'll cover this
depth in the 'Specific Goals' chapter. When it comes
re willing to sacrifice, I've supplied the rationale behind
and can't be consumed, along with some next bests for those
can't be consumed. What you decide to take, and leave, is up to
ou!

Fats

But first, fats. The effect of consuming fats whilst fasting is the cause for frequent debate. Consuming fats induces a minimal insulin response, and so you're still keeping insulin at bay. The ketogenic diet revolves around this idea of maintaining a low insulin state, consuming 80% of your calories from fat, 20% from protein, and limiting carbohydrates below 50g. You can picture consuming fats like 'flying under the radar' of fasting, with the primary benefits being a kick of energy or a feeling of satiation. However, it is important to note that they do break a fast, so if and how you use them really depends on what your goals are and the situation you're in. Me personally? I tend to steer clear of fats during a fast, I very much see them as a 'next best.'

A prime example of using fats whilst fasting is if someone just cannot do without their cup of tea in the morning, and definitely won't be having it black! Adding a small amount of almond milk or double cream to their tea, since both are largely made up of fat, with limited carbohydrates, can keep the effects to a minimum. You may also wish to draw out this ketogenic-like state once you do break your fast, refraining from carbohydrates until later in the day. I will note here that there's no need to get too caught up in some of these more advanced techniques, and everyone reacts to these macronutrients differently. The approach you take is very much down to you, your goals, and what you feel works best, manipulating fats is just another tool in your armoury to be aware of.

Terry Crews himself admittedly has "a little bit of coconut oil on a spoon" as a next best to feel satiated during his fast.

What Can't I Consume?

Many people state that you shouldn't exceed 50 calories during your fast, but to me that is misleading. You can't go ahead and grab half a banana and still be fasting; instead, these calories account for trace calories from what you may otherwise consume during a fast. For example: A cup of black coffee can contain up to 10 calories. In general, I recommend keeping it simple: Avoid anything with calories.

- Milk, creamer or sugar with tea or coffee. Next best: Full fat cream and almond milk.

- Teas containing fruit: Due to the sugar content - a bit of a nit-pick, if lemon and ginger tea is your go-to, I'll leave the ball in your court.

- BCAA's: A full serving of BCAA's contains roughly 50 calories, hence breaking your fast. Note the response incurred will be transient, so, if they work for you, you can decide if transient is enough to make you leave them.

- Vitamins with calories and oil capsules: Use alternatives if you can or take in the fed window. Otherwise, I wouldn't stress too much.

- Artificial and 'zero' products: The benefits of fasting could be interfered with by the consumption of artificial products, so I generally steer clear – unless your goal is simply to fast as a means of achieving a calorie deficit.

What Can I Consume?

Satisfying the want for consumption is a very useful tool to aid your fast!

I often find the simple process of consuming something, tea, coffee, even water, goes a long way in curbing the feeling when I'm experiencing hunger. There are specific goals, such as providing complete gut rest, where you may want to limit drinks, such as tea and coffee, and I will cover this point shortly. But, as a whole, the list provided below are all good-to-go!

- Water, and lots of it: Hydration is key when fasting.

- Sparkling water: Can suppress hunger. Personally, I don't overdo.

- Black tea and herbal teas.

- Apple cider vinegar: No calories, and a quick tip - diluting 2 tablespoons with water and sipping before your first high carb meal can stabilise blood sugar and further increase insulin sensitivity.[32][33]

- Salt: Sodium is vital for staying hydrated, and lowering your insulin can deplete your body of sodium - which can seemingly make you feel worse for wear. Consider adding some salt, maybe Himalayan, to your water. This won't break your fast.

- Toothpaste: Seems minor but worth mentioning. In my opinion, not something that's worth your energy worrying over. Go ahead and brush your teeth!

- CBD oil: Technically, CBD oil will break a fast due to its fat content, which will need to be metabolised. Therefore, it shouldn't be consumed for gut rest, however, for overall health, fat loss, cognition and longevity, you are good to go!

Black coffee, the first thing people recommend you consume outside your fast. You may wonder why this is separate from the list, and it's because a little more light needs to be shed. Black coffee can be consumed in your fast, the polyphenols in coffee can actually encourage autophagy, likewise with the caffeine it contains.[34] The caffeine can promote fat burning in a fasted state. Black coffee can also serve as a great hunger suppressant.

However, it's often overused. The overconsumption of coffee amps up cortisol, the stress hormone. This, when coupled with a period of fasting, can put you on a fast track to stress and irritability. Not only this but relying on coffee to get through your fasted period leads to dependency, caffeine tolerance and constant dehydration with it being a natural diuretic. Finally, drinking coffee on an empty stomach is a topic of great dispute. There is no doubt that coffee in excess can irritate the gut, and this can be especially the case on an empty stomach, i.e. when fasting.

Here, I would recommend caution and also consideration of the current state of your gut health. Also, noting that issues, such as leaky gut, can go seemingly asymptomatic in terms of the gut itself (no direct bloating or inflammation) but can cause issues, such as skin irritation and fatigue – prevent before you have to cure. Don't get me wrong; black coffee can be a great asset to fasting, just use it within reason, not as a sustained 'energy' source. Try switching it up with green tea, which also contains caffeine, along with the calming amino acid, l-theanine

Finally, another special mention can be made for bone broth! If we refer back to 'Gut Health', bone broth contains a host of vitamins, minerals and collagen, also containing high levels of anti-inflammatory amino acids that can help to heal the intestinal wall and aid those with digestive issues such as IBS.[30][31] In my go-to recipe, you'll also find salt, in my case Himalayan sea salt, and coconut oil, which makes it the perfect next best during your fast. Although it would be considered breaking your fast, a flood of all these nutrients, including sodium and healthy fats, would be the perfect way to prolong your fast as a next best if you're struggling that day. It's also the perfect way to replenish your body after a period of fasting!

How to Break a Fast

After a period of fasting, your body is like a sponge, highly sensitive and ready to absorb what you put into it, which means that you can be strategic in how you break your fast! I want to preface this point by saying that how you break your fast does not have to be of upmost importance – if constructing a "perfect" fast breaking meal or delaying a macronutrient only puts the breaks on your day and causes unnecessary stress, then stick to easily digestible nutrient dense foods.

Your gut has just woken up from its period of rest and kicking things off with an easily digestible meal seamlessly gets the wheels turning again. Moreover, flooding your body with a meal rich in nutrients really starts the process of re-nourishment, as you mustn't forget... a period of fasting followed by a period of sufficient feeding.

If you'd like to get more strategic, then introduce carbohydrates as the day goes on. Limiting carbs in your first meal can allow you to maintain a state of low insulin, also combatting cravings, leading to a feeling of fullness from the consumption of protein and fat. This allows your body to continue accessing fat as a fuel source, which helps to maintain metabolic flexibility and improve your metabolism, as discussed in the weight loss and metabolism chapter. Additional techniques include breaking your fast with just protein, breaking your fast with chocolate, and finally, with an apple! However, these points are discussed in more detail in 'Advanced Techniques', and not covered in depth here, as I want to ensure they are seen as advanced and not essential!

> *"Through fasting, I have found a state of perfect health, a new state of existence, a feeling of purity and happiness."*
> *— Upton Sinclair*

FASTING PROTOCOLS

If Intermittent Fasting is something you want to implement in the long term, seeing it as a tool that can be used when it suits your life situation is the most sustainable option. The same method of fasting will not work for everyone, the same method may not work for a given person in multiple circumstances. The path to follow is down to you as an individual, in the current situation you are in. Through varying fasting frequency and duration, a full spectrum of possibilities can be developed, supplying something for everyone. I'll discuss further which protocols line up with specific goals in the following chapter, and a little later, I'll dig into the steps to take in 'Getting Started'.

Duration

To see the full benefits of fasting, I suggest a minimum of 16-hour fasts, allowing for sufficient time to enter a fasted state beyond the previously discussed 'post absorptive' period. The further you fast beyond 16 hours, the further you dig into some of the benefits, especially fat loss, cellular autophagy and the full range of mental benefits. I've listed some of the most common fasting protocols, which cover a range of fasting durations.

24-hour fast – O.M.A.D. (One Meal a Day)

Exactly what it says on the tin! The O.M.A.D. diet means you consume your daily calories in one sitting, usually allowing one hour for eating. In no way do I carry a bias towards this approach; however, I feel this is only one to follow if it seamlessly works for you.

20:4 – The Warrior Diet

The Warrior Diet, consisting of 20-hour fasted periods, is an intensive method of fasting often associated with great body composition transformations, and through my personal experience, a noticeable mental clarity. In my opinion, it's great to take you to that next level, even if followed temporarily, best for experienced individuals who are already well adapted to fasting.

18:6 - My Fasted Lifestyle

This seems to get lost between the Warrior and Leangains, but it's my personal favorite! An 18-hour fast gives you sufficient time to explore the benefits of fasting beyond just body composition, whilst still being a manageable and potentially sustainable schedule for eating. I usually go for 2:00pm – 8:00pm!

16:8 – The Leangains Method

The Leangains Method is by far the most popular and well known method of fasting. To those new to fasting, this is a perfect starting point. I followed this approach for nearly two years when I first began fasting, eating from 2:00-10:00pm every day (the lateness isn't ideal on paper, but it was sustainable for me at the time!). When it comes to the social cost of fasting, this is also where you may seek comfort. With sufficient time to eat an early lunch, or even a late breakfast, still finishing up well into the evening. Definitely one for anyone looking to test the water with fasting.

12:12 – The Crescendo Method, up to 16:8

So you've given fasting a shot, but it still just isn't quite for you. The crescendo method is a protocol that allows you to consume all of your calories in a 12-hour window, say, 8am to 8pm. Although I wouldn't consider this to be Intermittent Fasting, there are still benefits to be had from not eating around the clock. This also applies to any other fasted period up to 16 hours.

Frequency

By altering how often you fast, you can tap into the benefits you're seeking and keep the intensity of the process where you'd like it to be. For example, you may want to fast for 24 hours for gut rest, with this being a lengthy fast, you may opt to do this just once a week, or even once a month. The less experienced you are, the less frequently you may like to fast whilst you adjust to the process. I will note, however, that fasting every day, within the same window, allows you to really take advantage of the adaptation that you will experience, especially when it comes to hunger. But, once again, it comes down to you as an individual and what you're looking to achieve.

Fast every day

Fasting is definitely something that can be done every day, speaking from experience, I find the best results come from a prolonged period of daily fasting. This removes the continual need to adapt to a new eating pattern and means you can really form a habit of fasting.

Fast every day, except when it's simply better not to

Brunch with an old friend, a weekend wedding, a holiday... don't let the process tie you down. If you want to squeeze in a late gym session, throw that protein shake down you at 11pm and keep the train rolling.

Alternate day fasting

One day on, one day off! This method never keeps you far from comfort, and that might be just what you need to form a sustainable lifestyle of fasting.

Fast a given number of days a week

Set yourself a target to fast a certain number of days a week, ticking them off on the days that work best. (Less advised, as you may just keep pushing it back)

Only fast on particular days of the week

Fast throughout the week and take the weekend off. Or vice versa, only fast on the weekends!

One long fast (24 hours for example) every week (or two weeks, or month...)

As simple as it sounds. Each week, find a single extended period, say 24 hours, where you abstain from food. If you have an early dinner at 4 o'clock on Saturday, you can pick up where you left off at 4 o'clock Sunday, having sufficient time to eat on both days.

There are no bounds

I would like to mention that there are no boundaries to the protocol you choose. Just because a 19:5 performed 6 days a week with a cheat day once a week (e.g.) isn't specifically listed, that doesn't mean it's not your 'perfect protocol'. Try things out, experiment a little, but most importantly... find what is sustainable for you!

> *"I only eat once a day and it's at night. But I eat until I'm*
> *full, I eat as much as I want, and I really don't eat anything*
> *that you couldn't find, you know, 10,000 years ago."*
> *– UFC Champion Ronda Rousey*

SPECIFIC GOALS

The protocol that you choose and what you consume during the fasted period depends on your goals. Manipulating what you consume when you aren't fasting can also facilitate these goals. So, now that you have an overview of the different fasting protocols, I'll be getting a little more specific, taking a look at how to tailor intermittent fasting to a variety of goals that you may have. Do note, you won't find every possible example here, only those that I felt required more detail. In covering a broad spectrum of possibilities, I hope to give you a framework so you can tailor your own 'Fasted Lifestyle'.

Samples to get you thinking...

Gut Rest and Digestion

For this, I'll need to get even more specific. If you struggle to digest large meals, I would suggest a daily 16:8 protocol, which gives you sufficient time to eat multiple digestible meals. Alternatively, you may want to fast for longer but less frequently; one 20-24-hour fast per week allows you to give your gut sufficient, regular rest. If you are able to digest larger meals, longer daily fasts, say 18-20 hours, may be more suitable for you. A combination of the two also works great. As someone who struggled from gut issues, I found that a daily 16:8, such that I could still consume enough to minimise weight loss, as I struggled to digest meals, with a weekly or bi-weekly 24-hour fast worked perfectly. A final suggestion would be to have your fasted window earlier in the day to sync up with your gut microbiome!

I would suggest avoiding the milk and creamer alternatives and any artificial products. Tea and coffee are more of an open discussion, as some find that it helps to keep things moving, if you will (sorry), others may find that caffeine serves as an irritant. This comes down to the digestive situation you find yourself with. Be sure to consume plenty of fluids; bone broth is a great one here, especially when breaking your fast for a flood of vitamins, minerals and amino acids. Also, consider the recommendations provided in 'Gut Health', including fermented food, probiotics and prebiotics, and dietary fibre!

Cellular Rejuvenation, Autophagy

When it comes to autophagy, the longer you fast, the better. Autophagy is a response to the absence of incoming nutrients, where your body looks internally, metabolising weaker and unwanted cells. The greater the need to remove these cells, the more this process is allowed to occur. For daily fasting, you can go for as long as you feel works for you. Alternatively, if you struggle to fast for longer periods of time or feel that it doesn't suit you, you can implement less regular, longer fasts. As far as alternatives and artificials, it's a no go. The discussion is open on caffeine; some studies suggest that sources of caffeine (coffee in the study used) may actually induce autophagy.[34] Based on the current research, we can't be definitive on this point. Again, consume caffeine (especially coffee) in moderation.

Low Insulin Levels

For this point, I'd like to focus on what you consume when you aren't fasting. Breaking your fast with a low/no carb meal allows you to further delay the insulin response from consuming carbohydrates. Having your first meal resemble the ketogenic diet can be a great way to provide your body with the healthy fats it needs, with some protein, delaying carbohydrates until your next meal. Something like tuna, eggs, avocado and a drizzle of olive or coconut oil works perfectly here! You may also choose to follow a diet resembling the ketogenic diet, but I won't be digging into that here. As alternatives go, you're all clear on that front, double cream or almond milk in tea or coffee, maybe even a dash of coconut oil. You won't be strictly fasting; however, this may aid the process and suit your needs. You can also gradually remove these additions over time.

Brain Function

A very difficult area to provide specifics; I have had mixed experiences, but adaptation is the key point. If you are not adapted to fasting, irritation will override any potential improvement in brain function. So, I suggest seeking consistency with a daily fasting protocol, allowing your body the chance to adapt so your brain can function optimally in the fasted period. Once you become more accustomed to the process of fasting, I would experiment with longer fasts - on occasions; I've found an incredible state of flow in longer fasts, making them the most productive days I'll ever have; other times, I can't keep my mind off food. When those days come is very situational, in my opinion. Finally, you may find that caffeine or even healthy fats like coconut oil can assist you here. During longer fasts, coconut oil can provide energy to the body and brain, although this would no longer be strictly fasting.

Fat Loss

Fat loss takes time, and that's why I suggest finding a daily fasting protocol that you can maintain. Consistency is key here. Fat loss is about far more than calories; however, the longer your daily fast, the easier you may find it to achieve a calorie deficit. In my opinion, having a period of the day where you can completely call yourself satisfied with what you've eaten is one of the keys to sustainability, and restricting what you eat to a smaller window of the day makes this more and more achievable – all the while, you're experiencing the benefits of fasting. A period of fasting, followed by a period of sufficient feeding. Noting that there is a very big difference between fasting and undereating, as we know from Angus Barbieri!

Alternatively, you may find that reducing the number of days you fast, and altering the length of your fasts accordingly, is a more sustainable option for you. The only thing I'd like you to consider here is that your body has less of a chance to become accustomed to eating in a given window. When it comes to fat loss, there is far more scope for alternatives and artificials; in this case, I will very much leave it down to you. If consuming something is going to help you sustain this lifestyle, then I would say it's worthwhile. Finally, be sure to carry through the tips and tricks from 'Hunger', including foods for satiation and high-volume low energy density foods.

Muscle Gain

The overriding message is to ensure that you can consume a sufficient amount within the window that you've chosen in order to optimise muscle growth. Having a regular period of the day where you tap into stored energy allows your body sufficient rest to process the increased food intake, maintaining metabolic flexibility. Limiting the window in which you eat can also stop you from greatly spilling over on your calories, minimising excess weight gain; hence, why fasting has become strongly associated with lean bulking. The hormonal response to fasting, including increased human growth hormone, will certainly cater to muscle growth here. How often you choose to fast is down to you; however, I once again suggest daily fasting.

Get in Shape Without the Stress

Want to get in shape and maintain it without the overbearing pressure that it can sometimes have? Then my suggestion here is simple: find a protocol that works best for you, one that you can see yourself maintaining for, well, ever! The sheer process of fasting, along with regular exercise, can be all some need to maintain the health and physique goals they have, without the need to watch what they eat quite so much.

Icons of TV and film Nicole Kidman, Jennifer Aniston and Halle Berry all swear by a fasting protocol to stay in shape.

FASTING AND EXERCISE

Training in a Fasted State

The benefits of fasted training is a controversial topic, especially when it comes to fat loss. Studies comparing fasted and fed training in individuals following a 'regular' eating schedule with the same caloric intake, where fasted training was performed in the morning followed by a post-workout shake, found that although fatty acid oxidation is increased during fasted exercise, total fat loss over time is unchanged.[35] This shows that fasted and fed training has the same effect on fat loss when performed with a normal eating schedule, providing the same daily calories are consumed. So, waking up early to squeeze your cardio in before breakfast isn't going to have any advantage over performing that training later in the day, provided your net energy balance over the course of the day is the same.

When a similar protocol was performed in physically active men who were fasting during Ramadan, training after 15-16 hours of fasting, a great representation of intermittent fasting, the results differed slightly. Body fat percentage (BF%) in the fasted group decreased by 6.2%, but the BF% of fed remained unchanged during the whole period of the investigation.[36] However, in this study, caloric restriction was not controlled, and the fasted group reported a slightly lower caloric intake during periods of the study. Again, standing to reason that fasted training is not beneficial over fed training for fat loss, provided total energy balance over the day is the same.

To summarise, training fasted appears to have no benefit on weight loss if you consume the same number of calories as you would otherwise.

So, what are the benefits of fasted training? As displayed by the fasted group during Ramadan, performing fasted training can make finding a calorie deficit easier. Training dissipates hunger, so any hunger you carry into a training session soon fades away. Once you've completed your session, you will need to refuel, regardless of the food you ate prior, and so for those who trained fasted, they will have consumed less calories up to this point, facilitating weight loss. Training fasted can also be used as a method of lengthening your fast. If you train at the end of your fast, the session will carry you through what may usually be a difficult period to abstain from food. With hunger dissipated, you may have added an hour or two onto your fast with no extra difficulty.

When training fasted, you'll also be clear from any interruption from digestion. Once blood flow and energy towards digestion is removed, your body can be fully focused on supplying those resources where they are required for training. A key point to be aware of is that fasted training doesn't interfere with muscle development, having said this, it may be sub-optimal for growth. The same men who fasted during Ramadan, lifting weights after 15-16 hours of fasting, found that body composition wasn't impacted when compared to those who trained fed. In terms of performance, the study also found that both groups maintained their training volume and didn't report changes in how difficult these sessions felt; this can largely be explained by the hormonal response to fasting. Whether or not you train fasted may depend on how your daily schedule lines up with your fasting schedule. So should the best time for you to train be in your fasted period, then I hope this research reassures you that you can still train to a high level.

A final benefit of fasted training is increased metabolic flexibility. Fasting alone increases metabolic flexibility by allow your body to tap into and effectively use fat stores for energy. Extending this into a training environment, where the energy demands are higher, allows you to become better accustomed to accessing stored fat and using it for fuel. This is a point of focus for many endurance athletes as discussed shortly.

Can You Train in the Morning and Continue Your Fast into the Day?

In my opinion, this is more of an advanced technique… Say you normally break your fast at 2:00pm, you can train at 8:00am and continue fasting until your usual time and still reap the rewards of that session. Should you provide your body with the correct nutrition in your feeding window, it's not going to disappear overnight. Having said this, intensity and frequency most certainly matters. A taxing session, especially resistance training, should be followed up immediately with post workout nutrition, ideally in the form of a combination of protein and carbohydrate.[37] Moreover, frequent fasted sessions without surrounding nutrition should be avoided. For optimal performance and recovery, this also may not be the best approach. Note, this is a case where consuming BCAAs may be the next best alternative.

Still not convinced? Terry Crews trains early in the morning, continuing to fast until 2:00pm, and he seems to be hanging on to his muscle just fine... Light-heartedness aside, my aim here is just to break down some of the barriers you might have about the 'necessity' of eating immediately surrounding your workouts.

But What About Endurance Training?

As I've previously mentioned, fasted training has become an integral part of endurance training and competition. The 2018 Kona Age Group World Champion, who also set the course record in the event, Dan Plews, is an advocate of fasted training and claims that being able to utilise fat for fuel is an integral part of endurance racing. I am not an expert in the field of endurance; however, through my own experience and research, the following recommendations can be made here:

- Keep fasted workouts to a low intensity, so you don't overtax your body and immune system, integrating a selection of fasted and fed training, tending towards fed training for the intense sessions.

- Ensure that if you are training again soon after or require optimal recovery from the given session, you consume a post-workout meal with roughly between a 3:1 - 4:1

carb:protein ratio.[38] A perfect example of this would be a peanut butter jelly sandwich! For 1 slice of whole wheat bread, 1 tablespoon of peanut butter and half a tablespoon of all fruit jam, you should be just in the right range.

A Final Word on Fasted Training

Training fasted can be a daunting prospect, but it's important to keep in mind that your body is very well-designed to perform in the absence of incoming food. If you can break down the mental barrier, fasted training can become a great asset to your training. Like any new stimulus for the body, time to get used to it is to be expected. To ease through this period, gradually build up the intensity and frequency of fasted training.

Finally, please consult your doctor to ensure that you are aware of any hormonal imbalances or other health issues that may lead you to refrain from fasted training; this is especially the case for women. Practice fasted training at your own discretion and moderate the frequency, duration and intensity of sessions. I will discuss in greater depth the considerations that women should make in 'Getting Started'.

Training in a Fed State

The primary benefits of training in the fed state are optimal strength, power, performance (in some cases) and recovery. The body uses carbohydrates as a primary fuel source when it's available, as it can be used directly from the muscle. So, providing you don't follow a low carb diet, having carbohydrates surrounding your workout are going to be optimal for both performance and recovery. For those performing intense workouts, including endurance training, consuming food ensures you don't overtax the body and the immune system. One thing to keep in mind… In the feeding window, especially straight after breaking your fast, your body is going to focus energy processing what you consume. So, be sure to give your body time to digest this food, or it may hinder your workout more than help. As a general rule of thumb for carbohydrates, consume low glycemic-index 90 minutes before, and high glycemic-index closer to the session.

Remember, You're Not Bound to Fasting!

Hold on a second! Before you go… please don't get too caught up in when you train. Sessions at all times of day are beneficial and will help you become the best version of yourself. Look to tailor a lifestyle that works for you around your life situation. Not one that pins you to a protocol, causes you stress, and may cause you to leave fitness and health at the wayside. If you want to train in the morning and think food would be best, then don't fast that day, maybe also stop eating a little earlier that day for peace of mind. If you train late in the day and want to follow it up with a meal or a shake, do so and pick up where you left off tomorrow.

> *"There are many ways to get fitter, stronger and leaner. You shouldn't discriminate against any or strictly favour one. As soon as you do, you close your mind and limit your potential."*
> *– Ross Edgley*

94

MODERN DAY FASTING

Intermittent Fasting may appear to have been a natural way of eating in the distant past, but in the modern world, however, not quite so much. With an abundance of food at our disposal and research teams whose sole purpose is to tantalise your senses with highly satisfying and palatable foods, there is a huge psychological conflict in abstaining from food. The demands of modern-day life are also very different to what they've ever been, especially psychologically. Not to mention the social pressure to follow the supposed 'norms' of eating. When explaining to people that you're fasting, they may look at you like you have two heads. "Really? Surely that can't be healthy". Going against the social grain is never easy. I can tell you first-hand that defending your choice of lifestyle to others can become a little taxing. However, this cannot be a reason to leave it at the wayside.

How to Bridge the Gap

I have proposed a few tips here to help create an environment that supports your fasted lifestyle, should you wish to pursue it. Before we start, there are a few things to expect when you go against the grain with something like fasting:

- Many will not understand what you're doing and will discourage you as a result.

- The modern world doesn't cater to a lifestyle like this, so if at times your mind cannot resist the sea of temptation it's not your fault.

- The sooner you normalise the idea of fasting, the quicker you will find success with it. Remember, fasting is not crazy!

Satisfy the want for consumption

There are times when we go to open the fridge when we aren't even hungry, times we'll put the kettle on, even though we're not really thirsty, what we do really want is just some kind of consumption. Satisfying this want for consumption without breaking your fast is an extremely useful tool, whether you develop a love for green or mint tea, black coffee (moderately), sparkling water… it doesn't matter! Just having something that you can go to alleviates this need for consumption.

Stay busy and remove the cues

Keeping yourself occupied in the fasted period will keep food out of the forefront of your mind. This period is great for keeping your mind clear and focused on the task at hand, so use that to your advantage! Make the fasted period a time for focus and productivity. By removing food from open sight, you also remove the cue to eat. If every time you walk into the kitchen, your favourite cereal is staring you in the face, you're setting yourself up to fail. Remove the cues of eating so that during the fasted period, food isn't rubbed into your nose while you're abstaining from it. Cues lead to cravings. Out of sight, out of mind. You can also cue positive habits, like drinking water! Leaving a jug of water waiting on the table for you when you come downstairs seamlessly leads to a glass while you're there.

Give yourself time to adapt

I've talked a lot in the previous pages about this seeming need to 'pass through a period of adaptation'. This won't always be easy, but it will be well worth it! When you start out intermittent fasting, I would give yourself at least a month to really see significant changes. Give yourself time for hunger to subside, for your energy to stabilise, and for you to start enjoying the process. I've heard many say, "Anything that takes this long to get used to and makes you feel bad before you feel good can't be healthy!", and to that I would say, how long does it take to truly quit smoking, or drinking? And how did you feel when you first stopped? Smoking, drinking and breakfast are clearly not comparable – but the process of breaking the mould that your body finds comfort is difficult all the same.

Be cautious not to build an identity around fasting

When a choice of lifestyle makes such a positive impact on someone's life, as is often the case with intermittent fasting, it can become very easy to pin yourself to this new lifestyle and build an identity around it. So much so that you can close yourself off to the possibility that any other way of living could be better. Intermittent fasting may serve you well in certain circumstances, and not so much in others. If you're heading for a hike with friends and family, you might only get so far before you halt the group to get some food in. On this occasion, it may just have been better to have a light breakfast to set yourself up for the day ahead. Being open to all possibilities and never settling on one specific lifestyle allows us to be flexible, as life is ever moving and changing. Intermittent fasting is a healthy lifestyle, but not the only healthy lifestyle.

Suggestion: Reflect and review – Regularly ask yourself these kinds of questions: "Is this choice of lifestyle still serving me?", "Would eating a few hours earlier just make sense in the situation that I'm in?", "How is my relationship with both food and those around me due to this lifestyle choice?", etc. Checking in with yourself is so important with any lifestyle choice, and intermittent fasting is no different.

Don't tell everyone that you're fasting, just do it!

Trust me when I say they'll hardly even notice. If someone offers you something to eat, and you're fasting, say, "No thanks, I'm all good", or "I've just eaten thanks". Responding with "Sorry, I don't eat until 2:00pm" will yield a line of questioning that will quickly become tiresome. If you live with a partner or a housemate, I would suggest not forcing the idea upon them to follow suit. Let those close to you know what you're up to and do your thing. Eventually, people will stop thinking you're crazy; some might even follow suit in time! It's a great feeling when that happens. At this point, you may start to develop a group around you that follow a similar lifestyle, which can be great to bounce off – I just wouldn't expect nor force this to happen immediately.

Don't put a label on the diet you follow or the lifestyle you lead

By attaching a label to your chest with your choice of lifestyle, you almost put yourself in a camp that leads you to believe you shouldn't stray from a rigid set of guidelines. In turn, this makes you extremely inflexible, which is an enormous disadvantage in my opinion. If you decide to follow a fasting protocol, you may actually sway towards a happy medium, somewhere between avid breakfast eater and one-meal-a-dayer, and you don't necessarily need a name or label for that! Intermittent fasting can be a tool in your toolbox to be used as and when its best. There will be days where it's less ideal, and in being flexible, you can... just not fast on those day! The same goes for vegetarian, vegan, keto, pescatarian, etc.; although you may want to follow one of these rigidly, there is no real name for someone who tries to avoid meat but only eats it when the other options are less nutritious or if the meat is high quality or grass-fed and eats fish fairly regularly but as a whole likes to stick to plant-based foods. Maybe flexitarian? But it's not necessary to pin yourself into a category!

Building a great relationship with food – a modern day challenge

Many find that intermittent fasting helps to build their relationship with food; many also find the opposite. If you previously found yourself stressing over continual restriction, then having a period everyday where you can be more relaxed with what you eat can be beneficial. If, however, you find yourself spending the entire portion of the day where you are not eating thinking about food, even having given yourself the time to adapt, planning what you're going to eat later, looking at your watch, counting the minutes… then this may be a red flag. Consider the protocol you currently follow. Is it sustainable for you? Are you eating enough when you are eating? Does the time that you've chosen to eat really coincide with your day?

We put a lot of pressure on ourselves to use our 'willpower' when controlling what we eat. It cannot be underestimated the impact your choice of eating will directly have on your brain. If you are not eating enough, your brain will likely tell you in all sorts of ways to eat more. So, consider this if you can't take your mind away from food. Is there a logical reason that this is happening? I personally get a little tough on myself when I think too much about food, "What is wrong with me? I just can't get my mind out the fridge". Rest assured, after some time eating a little more, the feeling seamlessly slips away. Try not to fight physiology; instead, work with it, listen to your body and be sure to give it what it needs to function.

Intermittent fasting may also seemingly cater to disorderly eating, providing a healthy reason to go an extended period of time without food following a large meal, as an almost, 'punishment'. In this case, I think it's all about intent, and the mentality that you are carrying into a fast. Meals should not be seen as a reward for fasting, and fasting should not be seen as a punishment for eating. If you find yourself carrying this mentality, I would possibly consider if this is the lifestyle choice for you. In which case, there is still plenty that can be learnt and taken from the process!

> *"I'm not a good faster. My friends have visions of God, I have visions of hamburgers. The only time I watch the Food Channel is when I'm fasting."*
> *– Bill Johnson*

ADVANCED TECHNIQUES

How to take it that one step further... It's a fine balance between advancing your techniques and needlessly over-complicating the process of intermittent fasting. These techniques are not necessary to be successful; however, being aware of them adds another set of tools to your toolbox, to be used as and when you wish. It's important to consider how these advanced techniques will affect the full picture of your lifestyle. For example, introducing carbohydrates, one of the techniques listed, may have a small benefit, but should this cause you to wait around and delay meals to squeeze this technique in, this small benefit will be far outweighed by the added complication to your day. In the same way that supplements are best used to advance, not replace, a balanced diet, advanced techniques are there to supplement a solid fasting protocol. Just another set of tools in the toolbox!

Get super spongey

Fasting alone increases insulin sensitivity, meaning you're more sensitive to the nutrients you take in. Exercising also increases insulin sensitivity, and so too does dark chocolate! Consuming dark chocolate in your post workout meal "turns your muscles into giant sponges that will absorb and use anything and everything you give them." – an extract from Ross Edgley's 'The World's Fittest Book'.[39] So, should you consume dark chocolate in your post workout meal, you'll already be pretty spongey. Should you work out at the end of your fast following up with this post workout meal, now we're getting super spongey!

I usually add a sprinkle of 100% cocoa powder into my post workout shake as a convenient method to apply this technique. Or, why not try a microwave protein chocolate mug cake? For whey protein add 2 scoops of chocolate protein, ½ tsp of baking powder, 1-2 tbsps of cocoa powder and 120ml of your choice of milk to a microwave bowl and microwave for up to 2 minutes. I like it very runny so I stop the microwave whilst the brownie still slides easily when you tilt the bowl. This can also be made with some vegan proteins, however I've had mixed success so I suggest researching a recipe for your choice of protein! You can spice this up by adding a handful of frozen berries or even a square of chocolate at the bottom for a melted chocolatey final mouthful!

Apple extender

A personal favourite of mine, especially when on a cut… when the time comes to break your fast, break it with an apple. An apple will replenish the glycogen stores in your liver and give you a feeling of fullness to extend your fast, with its high fibre content. This may give you just what you need to string out your fast for an hour or two. You can also combine it with some dark chocolate to increase insulin sensitivity and supply a boost of caffeine! For those seeking a calorie deficit, this can be an especially great option.

Introduce carbohydrates throughout the day

Although I've already discussed this point at length throughout the book, I do consider it to be an advanced technique. I will preface this point by saying that everyone interacts with macronutrients differently, and so this technique will not work seamlessly for everyone. Maintaining a state of low insulin can be a great way to reduce cravings and keep hunger at bay. It can also further increase metabolic flexibility as you encourage your body to tap into fat for fuel.

Mimicking the meal composition of the ketogenic diet for your first meal can be a perfect starting point here, something like tuna, eggs, avocado and olive oil. Or a more convenient option might just be a protein shake! Should you be training fasted, a quick protein shake at the gym can draw you out until your first meal when you arrive home. Finally, I want to highlight once again that putting the brakes on your day to squeeze this technique in may be more hassle than it's worth. Find what works best for you in the current situation you find yourself in, maybe just keep this as a tool in your back pocket! Want to take this a step further though? You can always…

Go full keto

The ketogenic diet can go hand-in-hand with intermittent fasting, and I have found great success with the two combined. The diet is composed of 80% of your calories from fat, 20% from protein, and less than 50g of carbohydrates. You could write a whole other guide to the ketogenic diet, which I won't be doing here; however, I would suggest you only try this in an environment that heavily caters to it.

Extended fasting

Extended fasting covers fasts greater than 24 hours long. You may remember that in the early stages of the book, I used extended fasting as a concept to better explain intermittent fasting. Although it requires a different approach to intermittent fasting, a lot of the key information provided in this book carries over into longer fasts. I've included this point as a steppingstone for your own research into the ins and outs of longer fasts. Please note, this book is not a guide to these types of fasts.

"The doctor of the future will no longer treat the human frame with drugs, but rather will cure and prevent disease with nutrition."
— Thomas Edison

GETTING STARTED

So, you have all the information you need, maybe more than you'd ever need! How do you get started? Everyone's approach to getting started will be different; some may be able to dive in two feet first, others will take a period of adjustment; this is where you need to be your own personal expert. The overriding goal is to form a sustainable lifestyle, so you need to consistently check in with yourself and how your choice of lifestyle is affecting your mental and physical wellbeing, and also your relationship with both food and those around you!

First Things First

Determine what you're trying to achieve! What are you hoping to get out of this lifestyle change? Zeroing in on your goals allows you to line up your lifestyle accordingly, and once you have your destination mapped out, the right path or protocol to get there will be much clearer. So, grab a piece of paper or open up a note in your phone and get down what you're trying to achieve by fasting so that it's crystal clear. Or...! Head to page 116 and follow the template supplied.

Where to start? - Daily Fasting

A protocol resembling a 16:8 (fasted/fed) is the perfect place to start or make your way towards. In a very short time, you'll understand how fasting works and what works for you. From there, you can look to make adjustments according to how you feel. If you get started with a 16:8 protocol, and it quickly becomes apparent that a different protocol may work better for you, then make these adjustments straight away. Otherwise, I would recommend giving yourself at least 4-8 weeks to adapt to the process.

1 - Two Feet First

Gradually closing the period of the day that you eat may not be necessary for you. It may be hard initially, but your body has the ability to adapt very quickly. So, if you're comfortable with it, you can dive straight into it.

- Pick a set feeding window, roughly 8 hours long.

- Choose a duration to try it for, 8 weeks is recommended to give you the chance to adapt.

- Stick to it! This doesn't mean slip-ups aren't allowed, just keep it simple and seek consistency.

We all have a different period of the day that suits us best, not only dictated by our day to day activity but also by understanding what you need to keep yourself on track and what you're willing to sacrifice. There is a noticeable benefit to skipping breakfast over dinner, as cortisol peaks shortly after waking, which helps to mobilise fatty acids, glucose and protein from storage for use.[40] Dinner is also where our social interactions gravitate. However, if you are unable to skip breakfast, delaying it slightly and having an early dinner works just as well. You could even skip dinner if that's what works for you! On the flip side, eating too late can misalign the body with its natural inclination to sleep, and likewise, for our gut, that's steadily winding down. As a general rule of thumb, try to push eating 1-2 hours after waking and round up 2-3 hours before bed.

Here are some common examples...

The early bird - 8:00-17:00 (9 hours - looking to close over time)

If you're a big morning eater, or you find it easier not to eat later in the day, this is a great option. With early eating windows, extending beyond 8 hours might be helpful; you may find you can push this later or close the window at a later date.

Early enough for brunch - 10:00-18:00 (8 hours)

If you find that pushing breakfast until 10 suits your day to day life, this is a great option. By 10 o'clock, you could be up and running, having set yourself up for the day, then before you know it, "It's that time already?". With this method, the later evening will be free of food, which may work for you.

The allotted lunch slot - 12:30-20:30 (8 hours)

Are you someone, like many, who has an allotted lunch slot at work? This could make your decision a whole lot simpler. If lunch is from 12:30-1:30, breaking your fast at 12:30 gets you all the way to 8:30. Once you've adapted to the process you'll have a boundary free morning before work and ample time to spare later in the day.

The late-night craver - 14:00-21:00 (7 hours, my choice for a long time)

If you struggle with late night cravings, like I do, pushing your window later into the day will mean you can still satisfy that evening urge. If having a glass of wine or an after dinner treat by the TV is what you need to stay on track, then cater to this, make sure your window finishes late enough so you can do so. From my experience, having broken your fast this late, you may not need to eat for 8 hours. Why not 7 or 6?

Are you free of limitations?

If you have more free time and you're less distracted from food. I find that there's a point at which you've sufficiently fasted, but you start to feel agitated, when your mental energy becomes diverted to feeding yourself. There's a sweet spot just as this starts to occur, where you've identified that it's coming but haven't yet allowed it to detract from your day. This may be a great time to break your fast.

2 - A Period of Adjustment

Intermittent fasting isn't immediately suited to everyone, but don't let that hold you back! With any lifestyle change, a period of adjustment is to be expected, and for some, this process requires more attention than others. Narrowing down the window that you eat might require some sacrifices, including lifelong habits that you hold onto, which isn't an easy process. This is where diving in two feet first might not be the wisest course of action.

There are two ways to gradually transition to a fasting protocol, the first being to close the window that you eat over an extended period of time, and the second, to take some time to adjust away from any pre-existing habits using "next bests". The rate that you close the feeding window is very much down to you as an individual; making incremental steps starting with, say, stopping eating two hours before bed, followed by delaying your first meal hour by hour into the day, may be a great way for you to transition. To adjust away from pre-existing habits, such as drinking tea with milk in the morning, you may like to use 'next bests' to make this process a little more seamless. Try adding almond milk or a small amount of double cream into your tea or make occasional swaps for black or herbal tea. In doing so, you can mitigate the effects on your fast, and you won't have to make too many changes all at once!

Differences for Women

Research has stated that intermittent fasting may react differently for some women when compared to men. Due to their reproductive system, women are more sensitive to calorie restriction as a whole, experiencing hunger signals more strongly than men. For this reason, I would suggest women follow their intuition more carefully. If hunger signals ever get out of control, it may just not be the day to fast. Understand that this is a natural physiological response and most certainly not your fault.

Excessively low body weight in any case may disrupt the production of reproductive hormones in women, which have the potential to cause irregular periods, infertility and other health effects.[41] With intermittent fasting carrying weight loss potential, this could be a potential concern. It's important to note here that research shows clear links between this hormone production and calorie intake, but not with fasting itself. This is where it's important to distinguish the effects of fasting and calorie restriction, a point discussed in 'Common Concerns'. Ensure that you're carrying the right intentions when practicing intermittent fasting, potentially leaning towards health and wellness benefits as opposed to weight loss if you are concerned about these issues – hence, ensuring you consume sufficient calories.

For these reasons, I would recommend women consider a less intensive protocol and build up to the process of fasting more gradually. The perfect starting point can be 12 – 14 hours of fasting, also potentially fasting on fewer days of the week. The 'Crescendo Method, 12:12', with 12 hours of fasting, can still lead to a whole host of benefits, and this may just be what's sustainable for you. Fasted training should be practiced with caution, as should intensive training on fasting days. Avoiding consecutive days of fasting can be a great call here too, so never fast for two days in a row! Finally, women, I don't want to warn you away from the practice of fasting, but feel this information can provide you with the context to best trust your intuition! If you just need a little reassurance that fasting is tried and tested for women; in all religious fasting practices, such as Ramadan, women do partake!

Suggestions: Gradually build up to the process of fasting, starting with 12-14-hour fasts, fast fewer days per week or avoid consecutive days of fasting, limit fasted training or excessive training on fasting days. Finally, ensure you are consuming enough calories to maintain a healthy stable weight to avoid disruption to reproductive hormones.

Longer Fasts

As you get into longer periods of fasting, there is a little more strategy to be considered. Should you be following a daily 12:00pm – 8:00pm protocol, and you want to introduce a weekly 24-hour fast on the weekends, starting late afternoon or early evening on Saturday, say 4:00pm, fasting until 4:00pm Sunday, allows you sufficient time to eat on both days. You may like to add an hour either side on both days, allowing you to eat from 11:00am – 4:00pm on Saturday and 4:00pm – 9:00pm on Sunday. Fasting with this time schedule spreads the time that you fast across the evening and following morning, with sleep breaking up the two. There are also psychological considerations to be made when fasting for longer periods. Keeping yourself busy, staying hydrated and fasting with other people are just a few ways to ease this psychological strain. 'Letting the floodgates open once you break your fast', as discussed in 'Hunger', is especially prominent after longer

112

fasts. I would refer back to my suggestions in the 'Hunger' section, and also recommend keeping food light and easily digestible once you break your fast.

Cycling a Protocol

So, you're off and running, and you've got a handle on what fasting is all about, why not experiment a little? Cycling a different protocol for a short period of time before returning to something (potentially) more sustainable may be the perfect way to test the water! You never know, you might just prefer it. You can also cycle a protocol that lines up with a specific goal you have. For example, should you be looking to lean down a little, a 4-week 20:4 'Warrior' cycle could be what you need to shake things up a little. Should you find yourself in a stable situation where a protocol fits your schedule, why not give it a go? You could have a 'going abroad' protocol or an 'exam season' protocol... Mix and match, depending on what life throws at you!

Humans Are Adaptive

When first starting a fasting protocol, results will come thick and fast, but this rate of improvement won't last forever! The human body is highly adaptive, able to adapt to whatever environment we throw at it, and fasting is no different. Around 12 months into intermittent fasting, I could hardly remember what eating breakfast felt like, and my body had found a certain comfort in this new way of living too. Depending on how far you have to go to reach your goals, at this point, some may turn the screw and look to a more intensive protocol as a

113

means of keeping the momentum going. This will only yield the same result in time as the body continues to mould to its environment. This concept can be applied to your training too! If your primary source of training is running, and you run 50km a week, every week, in time, your body will be well capable of running this distance and will require much less energy to do so. In order to see the same improvement, you start to up your speed or increase the distance.

So, what else can be done? I've found three primary approaches to avoid settling on a given fasting protocol, and they go as follows:

1. Maintain a certain flexibility with your fasting protocol – Avoid following the protocol too rigidly. Consistently taking your first mouthful when the clock strikes 1 and putting down the fork at 9 o'clock sharp with meals distributed the same way with the same macronutrient composition every day will allow your body to settle very quickly. A great tip here is to trust your instincts and eat intuitively day by day. If you're feeling more hungry than usual and want to draw your fast out another hour, follow that instinct and eat a little bit more on that day. On the flip side, you may feel perfectly satisfied and don't feel the need to eat more, or you're sailing through your fast and don't really want it to stop, then don't! This is especially the case when following an exercise program, as there will be times when your body needs to repair and recover; allow it to tell you that and give it what it needs!

2. Take strategic breaks – Once every … take a day off, a few days off, a week off! I feel the best times to take these break

are when the opportunity seamlessly arises. When that breakfast buffet that's to die for falls into your life while on holiday, maybe it's time to take the week off?

3. Keep the body guessing by switching it up or cycling protocols – You can also line this up with your training. If you're looking to both gain muscle and lose fat, try following a 16:8 'bulk', where you eat more and train to facilitate muscle gain. Followed by a 19:5 'cut', where you look to maintain muscle and trim any remaining body fat off. Cycling through phases of bulking and cutting whilst strategically widening your feeding window when aiming to gain muscle can be a handy way to visualise putting the extra time for food to 'good use'.

Should you decide to take a break from fasting, the advice given in 'Tips for Stopping Intermittent Fasting' will certainly be useful.

Balance

Each day is a chance to wipe the slate clean. Should you steer off course, there's nothing better than a fast to hit the reset button before kicking on again. In the same way that you need a holiday from work to come back better, or a day off the gym to come back stronger, there will be times where you need to break the rules before coming back ready to go again!

"Don't change your life to suit your fasting protocol, change your fasting protocol to suit your life."
– Ben Smith

GET CRYSTAL CLEAR

I am doing this because…

_____

_____

_____

My primary three goals are:

1) _____ by _____

2) _____ by _____

3) _____ by _____

MY PROTOCOL

I will fast/feed for _____ / _____ hours.

I will fast _____ days per week.

I will start at _____, and finish at _____

I will follow this for _____ months / weeks.

I will build up to this in _____ weeks (0 for two feet first).

Once I have done this, I will

_____

_____

_____

Remember, sustainability is key – this isn't a diet, so what comes next?

For example: I will adjust my protocol to what's sustainable for me in the long term. Or, I will continue until I reach my goal, and then I will… Or, I will keep going because this is really working for me!

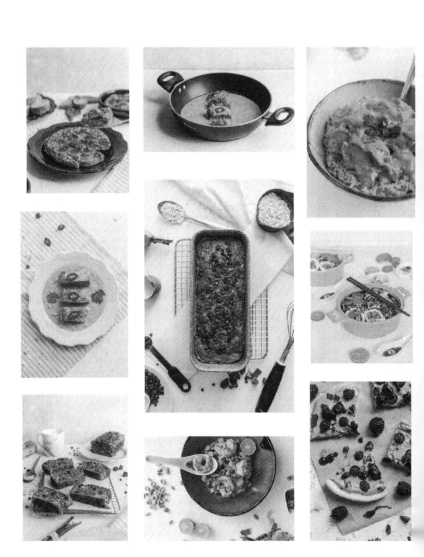

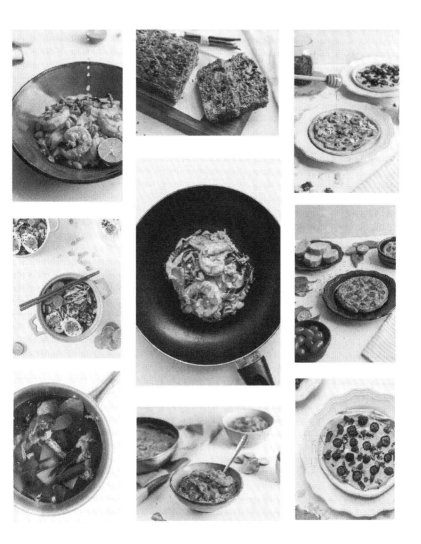

FOUR

FASTING CONSIDERATIONS

TIPS FOR STOPPING INTERMITTENT FASTING

COMMON CONCERNS

WHEN NOT TO INTERMITTENT FAST

TIPS FOR STOPPING INTERMITTENT FASTING

I don't mean to stop you before you even get started! Whether you're taking a strategic break from fasting for adaptive reasons, you just fancy some time away from fasting, or you feel it's not for you anymore, stopping intermittent fasting can be as tricky as starting it. Once again, you've become accustomed to a certain way of living, and reverting back may not be straight forward for everyone. So, I've put together a few tips to make the process a little bit easier, should you find yourself looking to take some time away.

Focus on the quality of food

When returning to an ordinary eating schedule, you may find difficulty in distributing your meals so that you don't overeat. Now that you're accustomed to a certain freedom with the quantity that you eat from fasting, this freedom may not be quite as prominent and that may take some getting used to. Some time to find your feet is to be expected, but my primary suggestion in the meantime is to focus on high-quality whole foods. Seek quality in what you eat as opposed to quantity, ensuring a balance of nutrients in each meal. You can also use some of the tips and tricks found in 'Hunger' to make sure you leave each meal full and satisfied.

Enjoy the process of making breakfast

After intermittent fasting for some time, you will be used to the early period of the day being free from food, and you may find the process of cooking, eating, cleaning, etc. a little stressful. It may feel like time's getting on in the day, and you're "still only eating". Making enough time so that you can relax and enjoy the process of cooking and eating makes this transition much, much easier. I can tell you this from personal experience. You could also consider prepping breakfast the night before!

Finding a happy medium

If you decide to stop or take a break from fasting, why go from one end of the spectrum to the other? There are lessons that can be learned from the process of fasting that can carry into a regular eating schedule. There's most certainly a balanced middle ground. If you wake up and aren't hungry or don't feel like eating, don't force yourself to; you're not "getting your metabolism going" by doing so. Also limiting late night eating, regardless of whether or not you are fasting, has major benefits to your health, so, now that you are no longer fasting, why not continue to cut eating off a few hours before sleep?

Follow an exercise routine – why not keep the fasted workouts going?

In the process of stopping fasting, there may be some weight gain concerns, and this is only natural. This doesn't mean, however, that the battle is lost! Focusing on a structured exercise routine can really add piece of mind that you're fuelling your training with this food consumption, supporting performance and recovery. Also, if you really hit it off with fasted workouts, why stop now? Fasted workouts may be another way that you can find that happy medium.

Avoid snacking between meals

You may have developed a habit of snacking in your feeding window when fasting, but with the new meal distribution throughout the day, this may be a great time to cut the snacks. By continually snacking throughout the day, you never allow yourself to fall out of that 'storing mode', as seen by a fall in insulin. Taking timely breaks between meals allows this to occur and also allows your digestive system to rest and get ready for the next meal. After eating breakfast, maybe try to visualise that you're still on your previous fasting protocol from that point, with your next meal being at 1:00pm (for example).

"If the only tool you have is a hammer, you tend to see every problem as a nail."
– Abraham Maslow

COMMON CONCERNS

If you need to take medication with food

If you are prescribed medication to be taken with food, I would recommend either of the following: Depending on the dosage, take in your feeding window if you can. Lengthen your feeding window to allow a greater spread of the medication across the day. Finally, don't fast on the days you need to take the medication, finding yourself a 'happy medium', as discussed in the previous section.

Alcohol

My approach to alcohol, and any food you might consume around it whilst intermittent fasting is very simple. Go out and enjoy yourself then wake up and continue on as if it were just another morning Except maybe now you'll need to focus on hydration a little more Continue fasting until your usual time and get straight back to it. Fo my first year of university, I followed a 16:8 protocol; any time I had drink or went over, I just acted like it never happened and didn't allo it to bother me nor make me stop altogether. This method worke great for me!

Separate the issues of weight loss from fasting

There are many health issues that can arise from chronically cutting calories and losing too much weight. Intermittent fasting can allow for ease in finding a calorie deficit, therefore, losing weight. And so, health issues can arise as a result of this weight loss or lack of nourishment, which are not directly linked to the process of fasting. These issues can be seen in a separate box related to the weight loss or calorie cutting itself, and so should be tackled separately.

Fasting does not have to result in cutting calories; it controls meal timing. If you are not able to consume sufficient calories to manage weight when intermittent fasting, I would consider if your feeding window is long enough, or if a full fasted protocol is the right lifestyle for you – remember, there are lessons that can be learned and happy mediums to be found! This discussion should be considered especially by women, noting the differences covered in 'Getting Started', as women react to calorie restriction with greater sensitivity.

Fasting's effect on thyroid function

When fasting, your body wants to conserve energy as it awaits the next arrival of food. This can affect thyroid function – especially if practiced too intensely, with too few calories consumed. The degree of caution that should be taken on this matter varies from person to person, but there are some foundational steps you can go through to keep your thyroid in check.

Firstly, ensure you are consuming enough selenium, iodine and zinc, which can be found in a variety of food sources or supplemented. These are nutrients that support thyroid function.[42] Secondly, avoid longer periods of fasting and chronic calorie restriction. This can be done by opting for a less intensive period of fasting, such as the 16:8, and ensuring you're consuming calorie and nutrient dense foods within your feeding window.

Moreover, thyroid hormones are produced in the gut, so properly managing your gut health is vital to thyroid function.[42] Gut issues, such as gut dysbiosis - an imbalance between the 'good' and 'bad' bacteria - and leaky gut can reduce T3 production. Finally, trust your intuition, especially with any stressful feelings, as stress and the resulting levels of cortisol can inhibit thyroid function.[43]

Overthinking and overanalysing

I'll be the first to say that I'm guilty here at times. It's very easy to slip into a state where you're stalling from one meal to the next. Waiting, watching the clock, thinking about the next meal before you finish the one at hand, "What should I have next?". This is often the case for me when I'm bored! Now, it's most certainly not always in our control; if you are not feeding yourself sufficiently, this thought will likely creep in whether you like it or not, so first and foremost, ensure that you're giving your body what it needs.

Finally, overanalysing how you feel and building associations between these feelings and the lifestyle you live and the food you consume can be problematic. Eating and healthy living are supposed to fuel your life, not encapsulate it. From my experience, I would recommend seeing the pursuit of healthy lifestyle in a complementary way, as opposed to the primary purpose of living.

"One must eat to live, not live to eat."
– Jean-Baptiste Poquelin.

WHEN NOT TO INTERMITTENT FAST

I am not a trained healthcare professional, and so I advise consulting your doctor before making any major dietary changes, like intermittent fasting. There are particular cases where this is most advisable, as listed below. Note, this list is not conclusive nor definitive. I also advise taking your own precautionary measures and doing your own further research before any kind of fasting, especially if taking any kind of medication or if you have any kind of health condition.

I would not recommend practicing intermittent fasting if:

- You are pregnant.
- You are breastfeeding.
- You have a health condition or you're taking medication that fasting may adversely effect.
- You are elderly, without consulting a medical professional.
- You have a history of disorderly eating or you feel like it increases or promotes unhealthy eating habits.
- You are underweight or have high caloric needs.
- You are under the age of 18, as you're still developing and have much greater growth demands.
- It just doesn't work for you.

CLOSING THOUGHTS

Why Did I Write 'The Fasted Lifestyle'?

In the ever-rising sea of information, intermittent fasting has made waves in the field of health and fitness in recent years. In the year of 2019, intermittent fasting was the most popular Google search relating to diet, an astonishing feat. What's come with this explosion onto the scene is a flood of information, and misinformation, on the topic. How could anyone possible sift through all this new research and advice? Well… that's exactly what I did. Along with four years of personal experience, I took a large sieve to all this information to create a complete guide to intermittent fasting, all in under 140 pages.

The fasted lifestyle has dramatically changed the course of my life for the better, and the purpose of this book is to provide such change in the lives of as many other people as I can. Even if intermittent fasting isn't for you, there are still lessons to be taken from the practice that can apply to any healthy lifestyle. Like any single tool, alone, it does not solve every problem. Dropping everything else you know about health and wellbeing or going to extreme lengths to fast when it would be better not to under the circumstances is only going to hinder your day-to-day life. This is where one of my favourite quotes from the book is particularly prevalent: "If the only tool you have is a hammer, you will see every problem as a nail." – Abraham Maslow.

FINAL WORDS

The final thought I'd like to leave you with is a phrase frequently used throughout the book: "Be your own best expert". I have had countless poor experiences with the healthcare system and many more poor encounters with misinformation online. One thing I've learned with certainty from this is that there is no substitute for your own intuition. No one knows you better than you. We are all biologically individual and interact with our environment differently, whether that be through the food we eat, the exercise we do, or the experiences we have. Question everything, whether that be articles online, advice from professionals, even the contents of this very book. I hope you found guidance and inspiration from this book and use it as a gateway to figure out your own perfect lifestyle, whether that be 'The Fasted Lifestyle' or otherwise.

> *"The fasted lifestyle isn't the only healthy lifestyle, but there are lessons that can be learned and practices that can be applied by everyone. Treat it as another tool in your armoury, an arrow in the quiver, ready to be used when the moment sees fit."*
>
> - Ben Smith

Thank you for reading!

Did **THE FASTED LIFESTYLE** meet your expectations? Want to help me ensure it finds the right people's hands? One **ENORMOUS** way you can do this is by leaving an **HONEST REVIEW ON AMAZON**. Everyone's review is read and very much appreciated, and honesty ensures the book finds those who will really take value from it! This can be done via the "Write a customer review" button at the bottom of the Amazon product page.

If you would like to connect with me head over to my Instagram @bensmithlive, I hope to catch up with you there soon!

To share your experiences following the reading of this book, feel free to email me at bensmithlive.uk@gmail.com for testimonials.

Be sure to use the hashtag **#TheFastedLifestyle** for any social media posts!

threemail.
brought to you by bensmithlive.

Have you ever suffered from ill-health, stress, low energy, brain fog, or lack of motivation, and can't seem to find a solution? Or maybe you're looking to make positive lifestyle changes for that new razor edge…

For some time now I've craved and searched for the seamless changes that lead to optimal health, living, learning and more – as someone who was never dealt the best hand in these areas, especially health.

I've created an intimate platform to share these ideas, thoughts and concepts, with those who are open and interested in them! It's called the **threemail.** newsletter, and the format is simple.

1 email, 3 new ideas, every week.

You can sign up at: www.bensmithlive.com/threemail

Sign up and join the inner circle!

REFERENCES

Over 40 cited scientific studies

1. Leah M. Kalm and Richard D. Semba (2005). 'They Starved So That Others Be Better Fed: Remembering Ancel Keys and the Minnesota Experiment', The Journal of Nutrition, 135(6), p1347-52. Available at: https://academic.oup.com/jn/article/135/6/1347/4663828

2. Stewart WK and Fleming LW (1973). 'Features of a successful therapeutic fast of 382 days' duration', Postgraduate Medical Journal, 49, p203-9. Available at: https://pmj.bmj.com/content/49/569/203.short

3. de Cabo, R. and M. P. Mattson (2019). 'Effects of Intermittent Fasting on Health, Aging, and Disease', New England Journal of Medicine, 381(26), p2541-51. Available at: https://www.nejm.org/doi/full/10.1056/NEJMra1905136

4. Natalucci G, Riedl S, Gleiss A, Zidek T, Frisch H (2005). 'Spontaneous 24-h ghrelin secretion pattern in fasting subjects: maintenance of a meal-related pattern', Eur J Endocrinol, 152(6), p845-50. Available at: https://pubmed.ncbi.nlm.nih.gov/15941923/

5. Jeff Rothschild, Kristin K Hoddy, Pera Jambazian, Krista A Varady (2013). 'Time-restricted feeding and risk of metabolic disease: a review of human and animal studies', Nutrition Reviews, 72(5), p308–318. Available at: https://academic.oup.com/nutritionreviews/article/72/5/308/1933482

6. Sutton EF, Beyl R, Early KS, Cefalu WT, Ravussin E, Peterson CM (2018). 'Early Time-Restricted Feeding Improves Insulin Sensitivity, Blood

Pressure, and Oxidative Stress Even without Weight Loss in Men with Prediabetes', Cell Metab, 27(6), p1212-21. Available at: https://www.ncbi.nlm.nih.gov/pmc/articles/PMC5990470/

7. Horne BD, Muhlestein JB, Lappé DL, May HT, Carlquist JF, Galenko O, Brunisholz KD, Anderson JL (2013). 'Randomized cross-over trial of short-term water-only fasting: metabolic and cardiovascular consequences', Nutr Metab Cardiovasc Dis, 23(11), p1050-7. Available at: https://pubmed.ncbi.nlm.nih.gov/23220077/

8. Johnson JB, Summer W, Cutler RG, et al (2007). 'Alternate day calorie restriction improves clinical findings and reduces markers of oxidative stress and inflammation in overweight adults with moderate asthma', Free Radic Biol Med, 43(9), p1348. Available at: https://pubmed.ncbi.nlm.nih.gov/17291990/

9. Alirezaei M, Kemball CC, Flynn CT, Wood MR, Whitton JL, Kiosses WB (2010). 'Short-term fasting induces profound neuronal autophagy'. Autophagy. 6(6), p702-10. Available at: https://www.ncbi.nlm.nih.gov/pmc/articles/PMC3106288/

10. Ganesan K, Habboush Y, Sultan S (2018). 'Intermittent Fasting: The Choice for a Healthier Lifestyle', Cureus, 10(7), p2947. Available at: https://www.ncbi.nlm.nih.gov/pmc/articles/PMC6128599/

11. Anton SD, Moehl K, Donahoo WT, et al (2018). 'Flipping the Metabolic Switch: Understanding and Applying the Health Benefits of Fasting'. Obesity (Silver Spring), 26(2), p254-268. Available at: https://www.ncbi.nlm.nih.gov/pmc/articles/PMC5783752/

12. Catenacci VA, Pan Z, Ostendorf D, et al (2016). 'A randomized pilot study comparing zero-calorie alternate-day fasting to daily caloric restriction in adults with obesity', Obesity (Silver Spring), 24(9), p1874-83. Available at: https://pubmed.ncbi.nlm.nih.gov/27569118/

13. Longo VD (2019). 'Programmed longevity, youthspan, and juventology', Aging Cell, 18(1), p12843. Available at: https://pubmed.ncbi.nlm.nih.gov/30334314/

14. Caesar R, Tremaroli V, Kovatcheva-Datchary P, Cani PD, Bäckhed F (2015). 'Crosstalk between Gut Microbiota and Dietary Lipids Aggravates WAT Inflammation through TLR Signaling', Cell Metab, 22(4), p658-68. Available at: https://www.ncbi.nlm.nih.gov/pmc/articles/PMC4598654/

15. Bhutani, S., Klempel, M.C., Berger, R.A. and Varady, K.A. (2010). 'Improvements in Coronary Heart Disease Risk Indicators by Alternate-Day Fasting Involve Adipose Tissue Modulations', Obesity, 18, p2152-9. Available at: https://onlinelibrary.wiley.com/doi/full/10.1038/oby.2010.54

16. Nørrelund H, Nair KS, Jørgensen JO, Christiansen JS, Møller N (2001). 'The protein-retaining effects of growth hormone during fasting involve inhibition of muscle-protein breakdown', Diabetes, 50(1), p96-104. Available at: https://pubmed.ncbi.nlm.nih.gov/11147801/

17. Anton SD, Moehl K, Donahoo WT, et al (2018). 'Flipping the Metabolic Switch: Understanding and Applying the Health Benefits of Fasting', Obesity (Silver Spring), 26(2), p254-268. Available at: https://www.ncbi.nlm.nih.gov/pmc/articles/PMC5783752/

18. Zauner C, Schneeweiss B, Kranz A, et al (2000). 'Resting energy expenditure in short-term starvation is increased as a result of an increase in serum norepinephrine', Am J Clin Nutr, 71(6), p1511-5. Available at: https://pubmed.ncbi.nlm.nih.gov/10837292/

19. Almeneessier AS, Alzoghaibi M, BaHammam AA, et al (2018). 'The effects of diurnal intermittent fasting on the wake-promoting neurotransmitter orexin-A', Ann Thorac Med, 13(1), p48-54. Available at: https://www.ncbi.nlm.nih.gov/pmc/articles/PMC5772108/

20. Newman, JC and Verdin, E (2017). 'β-Hydroxybutyrate: A Signaling Metabolite', Annual Review of Nutrition, 37(1), p51-76. Available at: https://www.annualreviews.org/doi/abs/10.1146/annurev-nutr-071816-064916

21. Bathina S, Das UN (2015). 'Brain-derived neurotrophic factor and its clinical implications', Arch Med Sci, 11(6), p1164-78. Available at: https://www.ncbi.nlm.nih.gov/pmc/articles/PMC4697050/

22. Espelund U, Hansen TK, Højlund K, et al (2005). 'Fasting unmasks a strong inverse association between ghrelin and cortisol in serum: studies in obese and normal-weight subjects', J Clin Endocrinol Metab, 90(2), p741-6. Available at: https://pubmed.ncbi.nlm.nih.gov/15522942/

23. Bastani A, Rajabi S, Kianimarkani F. The Effects of Fasting During Ramadan on the Concentration of Serotonin, Dopamine, Brain-Derived Neurotrophic Factor and Nerve Growth Factor. Neurol Int. 2017;9(2):7043. Published 2017 Jun 23. - https://www.ncbi.nlm.nih.gov/pmc/articles/PMC5505095/

24. Shariatpanahi ZV, Shariatpanahi MV, Shahbazi S, Hossaini A, Abadi A (2008). 'Effect of Ramadan fasting on some indices of insulin resistance and components of the metabolic syndrome in healthy male adults', Br J Nutr, 100(1), p147-51. Available at: https://pubmed.ncbi.nlm.nih.gov/18053308/

25. Shreiner AB, Kao JY, Young VB (2015). 'The gut microbiome in health and in disease', Curr Opin Gastroenterol, 31(1), p69-75. Available at: https://www.ncbi.nlm.nih.gov/pmc/articles/PMC4290017/

26. Fetissov, S (2017). 'Role of the gut microbiota in host appetite control: bacterial growth to animal feeding behaviour', Nat Rev Endocrinol, 13, p11–25. Available at: https://www.nature.com/articles/nrendo.2016.150

27. Cignarella F, Cantoni C, Ghezzi L, et al (2018). 'Intermittent Fasting Confers Protection in CNS Autoimmunity by Altering the Gut Microbiota', Cell Metab, 27(6), p1222- 35. Available at: https://pubmed.ncbi.nlm.nih.gov/29874567/

28. Del Chierico F, Vernocchi P, Dallapiccola B, Putignani L (2014). 'Mediterranean diet and health: food effects on gut microbiota and disease control', Int J Mol Sci, 15(7), p11678-99. Available at: https://www.ncbi.nlm.nih.gov/pmc/articles/PMC4139807/

29. Herbert T and Kaser A (2011). 'Gut microbiome, obesity, and metabolic dysfunction', J Clin Invest, 121(6), p2126-32. Available at: https://www.jci.org/articles/view/58109

30. Achamrah N, Déchelotte P, Coëffier M (2017). 'Glutamine and the regulation of intestinal permeability: from bench to bedside', Curr Opin Clin Nutr Metab Care, 20(1), p86-91. Available at: https://pubmed.ncbi.nlm.nih.gov/27749689/

31. Liu Y, Wang X, Hu CA (2017). 'Therapeutic Potential of Amino Acids in Inflammatory Bowel Disease', Nutrients, 9(9), p920. Available at: https://www.ncbi.nlm.nih.gov/pmc/articles/PMC5622680/

32. Petsiou EI, Mitrou PI, Raptis SA, Dimitriadis GD (2014). 'Effect and mechanisms of action of vinegar on glucose metabolism, lipid profile, and body weight', Nutr Rev, 72(10), p651-61. Available at: https://pubmed.ncbi.nlm.nih.gov/25168916/

33. Johnston, C, Kim, C and Buller, A (2003). 'Vinegar Improves Insulin Sensitivity to a High-Carbohydrate Meal in Subjects With Insulin Resistance or Type 2 Diabetes', Diabetes Care, Online, 27(1), p281-2. Available at: https://care.diabetesjournals.org/content/27/1/281

34. Pietrocola F, Malik SA, Mariño G, et al (2014). 'Coffee induces autophagy in vivo', Cell Cycle, 13(12), p1987-94. Available at: https://www.ncbi.nlm.nih.gov/pmc/articles/PMC4111762/

35. Schoenfeld BJ, Aragon AA, Wilborn CD, Krieger JW, Sonmez GT (2014). 'Body composition changes associated with fasted versus non-fasted aerobic exercise', J Int Soc Sports Nutr, 11(1), p54. Available at: https://pubmed.ncbi.nlm.nih.gov/25429252/

36. Trabelsi K, Stannard SR, Ghlissi Z, et al (2013). 'Effect of fed- versus fasted state resistance training during Ramadan on body composition and selected metabolic parameters in bodybuilders', J Int Soc Sports Nutr, 10(1), p23. Available at: https://www.ncbi.nlm.nih.gov/pmc/articles/PMC3639860/

37. Aragon AA, Schoenfeld BJ (2013). 'Nutrient timing revisited: is there a post-exercise anabolic window?', J Int Soc Sports Nutr, 10(1), p5. Available at: https://www.ncbi.nlm.nih.gov/pmc/articles/PMC3577439/

38. Ivy JL, Goforth HW Jr, Damon BM, McCauley TR, Parsons EC, Price TB (2002). 'Early postexercise muscle glycogen recovery is enhanced with a carbohydrate-protein supplement', J Appl Physiol, 93(4), p1337-44. Available at: https://pubmed.ncbi.nlm.nih.gov/12235033/

39. Edgley, R, (2018). The World's Fittest Book, Sphere, p163.

40. Lugavere, M and Grewal, P (2018). Genius foods: become smarter, happier, and more productive, while protecting your brain for life, Harper Collins, Ch. 7

41. Meczekalski B, Katulski K, Czyzyk A, Podfigurna-Stopa A, Maciejewska-Jeske M (2014). 'Functional hypothalamic amenorrhea and its influence on women's health'. J Endocrinol Invest, 37(11), p1049-56. Available at: https://pubmed.ncbi.nlm.nih.gov/25201001/

42. Knezevic J, Starchl C, Tmava Berisha A, Amrein K (2020). 'Thyroid-Gut Axis: How Does the Microbiota Influence Thyroid Function?', Nutrients 12(6), p1769. Available at: https://www.ncbi.nlm.nih.gov/pmc/articles/PMC7353203/

43. R. Malik, H. Hodgson (2002). 'The relationship between the thyroid gland and the liver', QJM: An International Journal of Medicine, 95(9), p559–69. Available at: https://academic.oup.com/qjmed/article/95/9/559/1574610

44. Fung, J and Moore, J (2016). The Complete Guide to Fasting: Heal Your Body Through Intermittent, Alternate-Day and Extended Fasting, Victory Belt.

An enormous thank you to the following people who helped to make this book what it is now!

Recipe images: Arianna Martínez

Cover formatting assistance: Zeeshan Alam

Editing assistance: Michele Berner

Internal formatting assistance: Ehtisham Altaf

Printed in Great Britain
by Amazon

63097755R00086